S0-BSD-634

365 WAYS TO
Look–and Feel–
younger

Easy Solutions to Turn Back the Clock

Everyday Tips to Reduce Wrinkles, Improve Memory, Boost Libido, Build Muscle, and more!

MEERA LESTER AND CAROLYN DEAN, MD

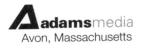

A adamsmedia
Avon, Massachusetts

I dedicate this book to my husband Carlos Jose Carvajal,
whose love and support keep my spirit young, my heart strong, my brain sharp,
and my dancing feet ever in motion.

Copyright © 2010 by F+W Media, Inc.
All rights reserved.
This book, or parts thereof, may not be reproduced in any form without permission from the
publisher; exceptions are made for brief excerpts used in published reviews.

Published by
Adams Media, a division of F+W Media, Inc.
57 Littlefield Street, Avon, MA 02322. U.S.A.
www.adamsmedia.com

ISBN 10: 1-4405-0222-6
ISBN 13: 978-1-4405-0222-4

Printed in the United States of America.

10 9 8 7 6 5 4 3 2 1

Library of Congress Cataloging-in-Publication Data
is available from the publisher.

This book is available at quantity discounts for bulk purchases.
For information, please call 1-800-289-0963.

Contents

Introduction

How many times have you looked into the mirror and wondered what you could do about restoring that youthful glow to your skin, minimizing those crow's feet and laugh lines, and putting the sheen back in your hair? How often have you thought about losing the weight you've slowly been gaining, getting rid of your belly fat, strengthening and toning those flabby muscles, or getting back the sexual "va-va-voom" that you had in your early twenties? If you answered, "often," you are not alone. Millions of Americans, just like you, seek natural and healthy ways to turn back the clock—to look and feel younger than the image they see reflected in their mirror.

The good news is that much more is known now about the aging process, and research is still continuing. Just because you are getting older doesn't mean you necessarily have to suffer from diseases that in the past have been associated with aging. Why? Because it is now possible to separate aging from acquiring age-related disease, according to Dr. Andrew Weil, best-selling author and founder and director for Integrative Medicine at the Health Sciences Center at the University of Arizona. Maintaining good health is almost a skill set that can be learned.

This book contains cutting-edge information that sheds light on how the body ages and what you can do to stay healthy, sexy beautiful, mentally bright, and just plain happy throughout your life.

In addition, you'll learn how herbs, vitamins, and minerals can contribute in your effort to stave off age-related diseases such as heart disease, cancer, and stroke. You'll find tips on getting a good night's sleep, making healthy lifestyle choices, and indulging in frequent sensational sex with your partner. You'll gain insights into why it's important to have a strong social network, avoid contaminants and pollutants, and integrate meaningful and sacred elements into your life. You'll discover which anti-aging foods will keep you fit and boost your immune system. And finally, you'll learn techniques and strategies for banishing stress and boosting brain power.

Replacing an unhealthy diet and lifestyle with new foods and fun activities is a great way to start on the anti-aging path. With this little book as your guide, you just might be able to shave off some years by taking back control of your fitness, your mental fortitude and agility, and your general health and well-being. Oh, and soon you can put that mirror away. You won't need it when people start asking you to share the secrets of your youthful appearance.

ACKNOWLEDGMENTS

I'd like to thank Paula Munier, who first brought me the idea for this project, and her team for bringing the book to fruition. I also want to thank Andrea Norville, whose skillful editing for content, clarity, and flow made the book immensely more readable.

chapter one
Save Your Skin

1.

Keep Makeup Cool to Preserve Its Integrity

Hot climates and extreme weather conditions during summer months can wreak havoc on ingredients in organic and natural makeup, causing oils and emollients to go rancid and other ingredients to be less effective. Try storing makeup in the refrigerator to preserve it. If you don't want to store your makeup in the refrigerator, find a cool, dry place elsewhere in your home to keep your beauty products as fresh and viable as possible. Makeup costs money, some items can be quite costly, so take the extra step to ensure that you aren't throwing money away and that the products that you are putting on your skin are safe and effective.

2.

Buy a Juicer

Can you say antioxidants? During a crisis, your body responds by releasing turbo-charging stress hormones that flood your cardiovascular system to prepare you to deal with the emergency. But stress hormones flooding the system can also cause damage. Antioxidants, substances found in certain fruits and vegetables, act as scavengers of free radicals (by-products created when cells use oxygen), and can both prevent and repair free radical damage. Your skin responds to antioxidant-rich nutrients that you eat, drink, ingest, and apply upon it. Squeeze or use a juicer to extract the juice from organic vegetables and fruits such as oranges, limes, strawberries, carrots, apricots, peaches, cantaloupes, and green leafy vegetables. Pomegranate, purple grapes, and cranberries are high in phytochemicals and are good antioxidant agents as well.

3. Take Vitamin C to Fight Free Radical Damage

The activity of free radicals (unbalanced oxygen molecules containing an extra electron that are constantly searching for molecules to which they can attach and steal a matching electron) is necessary for hormone synthesis, smooth-muscle tone, and the maintenance of a strong immune system as well as great-looking skin. Problems occur when free radicals attack cell membranes, inhibiting the cells' ability to reproduce or protect themselves. The effects of too many free radicals include some of the better-known signs of aging—wrinkles, age spots, and poor skin quality. An abundance of free radicals can also lead to cataracts, heart disease, and even the formation of certain kinds of cancer. Anti-aging researchers say that the answer can be found in chemicals known as antioxidants, which eat up excess free radicals. Vitamin C, taken as a supplement and also used topically on the skin can help protect against damage caused by free radicals.

4. Use Natural and Organic Makeup

The use of natural and organic products, including makeup, is on the rise. Mineral makeup products that rely on finely ground minerals, such as mica, titanium dioxide, and zinc oxide for blushes and powder foundations are hugely popular. Many women feel that the lack of fragrance, dyes, binders, and preservatives in mineral makeup makes these products kinder to the skin than traditional makeup. Locate numerous sources for organic, natural cosmetics, many from green companies, at *www.greenpeople.org/OrganicSkinCare.html*.

5. Slather on Sunscreen with SPF 15 or Higher

To avoid the risk of skin cancer, get used to applying sun screen daily before your makeup and reapply often when swimming. The sun's harmful ultraviolet rays are your skin's worst enemy. The Centers for Disease Control (CDC) recommends applying sunscreen liberally at least thirty minutes before exposure to the sun. By liberally, the CDC suggests a full ounce, or roughly a handful, to cover your body. Also, the CDC advocates choosing a broad-spectrum sunscreen that offers a sun protection factor (SPF) of at least 15 and protects against both the UV-A and UV-B rays. If you have acne breakouts or will be sweating or swimming, you might want to purchase a sunscreen that is waterproof. Check expiration dates as well because ingredients in sunscreen products can degrade over time.

6. Get a TCA Skin Peel

Although the trichloroacetic acid (TCA) skin peel is available as a nonprescription item, it is always prudent to consult with your dermatologist or esthetician first to discuss the pros and cons of having the peel, whether or not you are a good candidate for the peel, and if your skin might best benefit from a light or deep peel. The TCA skin peel is effective for minimizing or erasing acne, age spots, dull skin, wrinkles, freckles, scarring, and uneven pigmentation. Typically, your doctor will carefully apply the solution to your face like an astringent, avoiding eyes and lips. Your skin will feel and look like you've just had a sunburn. By the next day, it will begin to turn darker and feel tight. Subsequently, the peeling will begin and last for up to a week. Your new skin will emerge looking more radiant, fresh, and younger.

7. Use Baby Oil to Seal in Moisture

Moisturizing your skin is one of the most important things you can do to keep it looking young and fresh. Keeping your skin moisturized will pay big dividends in helping you stay great looking at every age. Some moisturizers act as a sealant, trapping the water in your skin. Others actually release water or moisture into the skin. It is important to choose a natural moisturizer, free of dyes, harsh additives, and perfumes. An inexpensive moisturizer is baby oil. Try rubbing small amounts into your skin after a warm shower before you have dried your body with a towel. Or, wash your skin gently and pat it partially dry and then immediately apply a moisturizing cream or lotion.

8. Take a Sauna or Steam Bath

If you want glowing skin, try a sauna (dry heat) or a steam bath. Taking a sauna or steam bath can eliminate toxins and excess sodium, relax tense and sore muscles, and enable you to ease into your happy place. If you want to build your own sauna or steam bath, kits are available online at www.saunas-n-sauna-kits.com/steam_sauna.htm. Or, create a mini steam bath for your face by simply boiling water in a pan or teapot. Pour it into a glass or ceramic bowl. Drape a bath towel over your head to form a tent and then lower your face toward the bowl. This tent contains the steam. Allow the steam to penetrate your skin for ten to fifteen minutes. For a little aromatherapy, add a few drops of your favorite essential oil or allow some fresh herbs to infuse the water. Drink lots of water to replace what you lose from the heat.

9. Make Your Own All-Natural Mask from an Egg Yolk and Honey

Ever heard of using cucumber slices to soothe and reduce puffiness around the eyes? How about lemon juice as an astringent for oily skin, or apple cider vinegar to rinse soap from your hair and add shine? Some of the skin and hair products our mothers and grandmothers used contained only natural ingredients they could find in the kitchen. Consider trying them. Make a facial mask with one egg yolk mixed with honey. Gently spread the mixture over your face after washing it with warm water. Wait about a half hour, and then wipe it off with a warm wet washcloth, followed by a cool water rinse. To get a clean, tight feeling, spread a well-beaten egg white (not the yolk) onto your face, let it dry, and then rinse. Or try a mixture of olive oil and kosher salt or sea salt to make an all-natural scrub. Just mix one tablespoon of oil to three tablespoons salt.

10. Eat Blueberries and Other Nutrient-Rich, High-Fiber Fruits

Dermatologists will tell you that beautiful skin starts on the inside with the nutrients that you consume, as well as sufficient water and juices high in antioxidants. Fruit is full of healthy substances such as vitamin C, vitamin A, potassium, folic acid, antioxidants, phytochemicals, and fiber, to name a few nutrients beneficial to great-looking skin. Citrus fruits, melons, and berries are excellent sources of vitamin C. When it comes to fruit, apples, bananas, berries, citrus fruit, and melons are your best bets because of their high fiber and nutrient content. Be thoughtful about what you eat and whether it benefits or hurts your skin.

11. Get an Aromatherapy Massage

Get a massage if you are having trouble getting rid of the tension or if you seek stress or pain relief. There are as many different types of massages as there are spas that offer them. For example, you could try a hot-stone massage, a deep-tissue massage, a prenatal massage (a mother-to-be necessarily requires different positioning and may also need attention to her lower back) reflexology massage, a Swedish massage, or the ever-popular aromatherapy massage. Aromatherapy combines a fragrant essential oil such as peppermint, rose, sage, chamomile, sandalwood, or ylang ylang as part of the massage treatment to induce deep relaxation. When warm oil is massaged into flaky, dry skin, softer, smoother skin is almost immediate. An effective massage can reduce your respirations and heart rate and lower your blood pressure. With regular massages, you will feel great and your skin will look younger.

12. Stimulate Collagen Renewal

Collagen collapse causes wrinkles, sagging skin around the mouth and neck, pucker lines along the lips, and fine lines as well as deep creases along the forehead, between the brows, and elsewhere on the face. But scientists at the University of Michigan say that certain treatments can actually stimulate collagen production. The results of their research and dozens of other studies affirm that topical retinoic acid, carbon dioxide laser resurfacing, and lastly, injections of cross-linked hyaluronic acid can stimulate new collagen. The collagen renewal from those treatments resulted in dramatic improvements in the appearance of the skin. Talk with your doctor about these treatments to see if one or more could help you recapture a more youthful face and neck.

13. Exfoliate with Sea Salt

Regular exfoliation of your skin produces healthier-looking skin and aids in the development of new collagen. The options for removing dead skin cells that dull your complexion include chemical peels, retinoids (products containing Retin A), microdermabrasion (usually done by an esthetician or a skin doctor) and a mildly abrasive scrubber. The latter may use ground grape, olive, or apricot seeds as the abrasive agent. Schedule a skin peel not more than every six weeks (the time it takes for the skin to renew itself). Estheticians say that you can literally turn back the clock several years if you just have regular peels. Alternatively, you can make your own exfoliating scrub using sea salt. There are a variety of recipes available on the Internet. Many start with one part oil (such as sweet almond oil) and two parts sea salt, which results in a somewhat thick mixture. You can add more oil to thin it if you like a more liquid scrub. You can also add other ingredients such as a fragrant essential oil or honey as a softening agent.

14. Read the Fine Print on Your Anti-Aging Skin Care Products

The packaging of many skin care products often touts anti-aging formulations containing collagen, elastin, vitamin A, vitamin E, keratin, retinol, and time-release nutrients, among various other ingredients. However, read product labels carefully to find out exactly what you are actually applying to your skin. If you are an allergic type, you might want to avoid skin products and makeup containing para-aminobenzoic acid (PABA) and other known allergens, which can trigger allergic reactions. Even the highly popular mineral makeup can cause allergies in some people. The most expensive makeup and skin care products do not necessarily equate with being the safest or the best. Check ingredients listed in the fine print before jumping on the bandwagon of the latest and greatest anti-aging beauty product.

15. Treat Yourself to Thassalotherapy

Increasingly, day spas, health spas, resorts, and even some cruise ships offer full-body treatments incorporating thassalotherapy—a spa therapy modality that involves a seaweed wrap of mineral-rich marine products, including sea water. But whether your favorite spa offers thassalotherapy, mud baths, or some other water therapy, you'll likely enjoy the break and gain a therapeutic benefit from your time spent there. The therapeutic use of water dates back to the fifth century B.C. and Hippocrates, the Greek widely known as the Father of Medicine. Although traditionally, hydrotherapy meant treatment with water of different temperature or form, such as ice packs and vaporizers as well as hot baths, modern spas generally use water to relax you while replenishing the moisture necessary for youthful, supple skin.

16. Get a Regular Facial

Estheticians in the offices of dermatologists and spas have been taught tricks and strategies to help you rejuvenate your tired skin and erase some of the fine lines and hyperpigmented areas (often the result of sun damage). A good esthetician will be able to identify your skin type and recommend a skin care regimen that's right for you. From simple facials to the more aggressive microdermabrasion or laser treatments, and chemical peels, estheticians can clean and revitalize your skin. They can wax eyebrows and lips, clean clogged pores, and guide you toward products that enhance your natural beauty. If you have spots or areas of hyperpigmented skin requiring a little lightening, your esthetician might recommend using some products that contain alpha hydroxy acids (AHA) or possibly ascorbic acid.

17. Visualize Yourself as Having Great Skin

Let your inner beauty shine. Do you see yourself as too wrinkled, thin, fat, disproportional, flabby, old, weak, frail, wracked with pain, or prone to illness? Such mental messages may or may not be true, but you can increase your sense of well-being, improve your health, and develop your inner beauty by changing negative thoughts into more positive messages, according to practitioners of the law of attraction. Your thoughts trigger emotions that can be negative or positive, so if you are giving yourself negative, critical messages, chances are you are neither looking nor feeling good. Conversely, if your thoughts are optimistic and you can see that somewhere inside you is a poised, healthy, energetic and beautiful person, you are more likely to be able to manifest that magnificent you.

18. Wear Cotton Gloves to Bed

Petroleum jelly and cotton gloves can work together to soften and soothe dry, cracked, or chapped hands. Petroleum jelly works as a great moisture barrier. Before bed, simply wash and rinse your hands. Pat dry, but not completely. Then, massage a small amount of petroleum jelly into them and slip on some cotton gloves. When you awaken in the morning and remove the gloves, you'll discover the skin on your hands will be much softer to the touch. This can also work for the feet. Be sure to use clean white socks after applying the petroleum jelly.

19. Treat Cracked Heels with Glycerin or Lanolin Cream

Cracks in heels that don't respond to daily foot care such as washing, drying, and using a pumice stone or rasp for filing off dead skin may require a more intensive treatment. The cracks, also called heel fissures, are often the result of dry skin and lack of attention to the daily wear and tear on your feet. Try a daily foot soak in warm water, then dry your feet and massage in glycerin or lanolin cream to soften the heel tissue. It won't be long before you'll be ready to show off those beautiful feet in sleek sandals or sling-back pumps.

20. Use Aloe to Treat Minor Insect Bites and Sunburns

Aloe vera is a succulent plant that contains a sappy liquid or gel that has been used as an effective topical treatment for minor sunburn, insect bites, and skin irritation and rashes arising from exposure to certain poisonous plants like poison oak and ivy. Aloe is an active ingredient found in numerous skin care products such as lip balm, healing ointments, shampoos, sunscreen lotions, and a variety of cosmetics. Grow an aloe plant in your home or outside if you live in a warm climate. To use aloe on your skin, simply cut off a piece of a stalk and apply the cut end (which will ooze with sappy liquid) directly on the skin. Although allergy to aloe is rare, if you think you are having an allergic response to it, consult your doctor.

21. Know the Signs of Skin Cancer

People with fair skin who easily sunburn, especially those with blonde or red hair, have less melanin in their skin cells and therefore may be at higher risk for the development of melanoma. This type of skin cancer is widely believed to be caused by exposure to the ultraviolet radiation of the sun. The Cancer Research Institute offers the following ABCDs of identifying melanoma:

A is for asymmetry. Melanoma lesions are not symmetrical, but rather irregular in shape.

B is for border. Melanoma lesions often have irregular borders in contrast with moles that have smooth, even borders.

C is for color. Look for brown and black color in melanoma lesions in contrast to moles that are often one shade of brown.

D is for diameter. Melanoma lesions routinely are about the size of a pencil eraser, roughly one-quarter inch or six millimeters across.

22. Get That Eyelid Skin Checked

Age makes us more prone to a variety of other vision disorders, including cataracts, glaucoma, diabetic retinopathy, and macular degeneration. Dry-eye is a common complaint among many older people because of diminishing tear production, and there may also be a wrinkling and loosening of the skin around the eyelids due to loss of tone and decreased elasticity of the eyelid muscle. In addition, a loss of orbital fat often causes the eyes to sink deeper into the skull, limiting upward gaze. If you have concerns about how your droopy eyelids may be affecting your vision, get it checked out by an eye doctor or plastic surgeon. Genetics may play a role in the appearance of loose skin around the eyes, but fortunately there are options for dealing with it.

23. Eat Cauliflower, Cabbage and Other Cruciferous Veggies

The link between good nutrition and great-looking skin is indisputable. Vegetables are packed with all types of healthy nutrients and some have antioxidant properties that could help slow aging of your skin. Daily requirements for several vitamins—including vitamin C, folic acid, and beta-carotene, the precursor for vitamin A—can be met almost exclusively from fresh vegetables and fruits. This is especially true with dark-green leafy vegetables, such as spinach or broccoli, and dark orange vegetables, such as carrots or yams. Some vegetables also supply sufficient amounts of calcium, iron, and magnesium. In addition to nutrients, vegetables also contain phytochemicals that may provide additional health benefits. It's a good idea to load your diet with as many cruciferous vegetables (such as collard greens, kale, cauliflower, cabbage, and others) as possible because of their cancer-preventing antioxidant properties.

24. Map the Moles on Your Body

One way to know where the moles and skin irregularities are on your body is to make a map. Why would you want to do this? Often the first sign of a skin cancer is a change in the appearance of a mole or a sore that doesn't heal. During your twenties and thirties, in particular, it's a good idea to get checked every three years for changes in your skin, especially moles. Although as a young adult, you may think you are infallible to the ravages of the sun, you aren't. Young adults engage in riskier behaviors than middle-age and older individuals and, because they often have an attitude that a tanned body looks healthier, they could be sowing the seeds for skin cancer to develop later. Making a map can be as simple as drawing a generic body and putting a dot on the drawing that corresponds to the mole and other spots you want to watch. You could also take photos in order to have a frame of reference for future examinations.

25. Understand What Cosmeceuticals Can and Cannot Do

As members of the baby boomer generation enter their fifties and sixties, an increasing number are turning to pricey "cosmeceuticals"—cosmetics specially designed to prevent or eliminate wrinkles and other age-related skin blemishes—in an effort to maintain their youth. Do these products work? Yes and no. They all contain essentially the same ingredients (antioxidants, copper peptides, moisturizers, hydroxy acids) but in varying amounts and combined with a wide variety of other ingredients. Many have been shown to eliminate fine lines on the face, but the effect is temporary and usually very subtle. Bottom line: Nothing that comes in a jar, no matter how much it costs, will get rid of deep wrinkles. For that, you need to consult a plastic surgeon.

26. Get Savvy about Skin Irritants

A whole pantheon of potential skin irritants in household products can manifest as skin irritations or dermatitis and bring on itchy bumps, weepy blisters, the dreaded hives, and other assorted manifestations of skin irritation. There are many substances that have been identified by doctors, scientists, and product manufacturers as skin irritants. If you have sensitive skin, you likely already know how unpleasant an episode of contact dermatitis can be. Read labels on products, including detergents, fabric softeners, soaps, and other household cleaning and laundry products for information about what, if any, skin irritants they contain. Look for environmentally safe products such as those by Seventh Generation that are nontoxic, hypoallergenic, and perfume- and dye-free.

27. Get a Vitamin C Facial for a Brighter Complexion

Vitamin C can almost perform a magic trick on your skin right before your eyes. If you seek ways of perking up your appearance, especially if your skin is looking a little dull or tired, try a vitamin C facial. There are quite a few skin-brightening facial products, cleansers, and hydrators on the market. Most say they do not dry the skin, but you'll need to test several to find the one that feels best to you. Use a skin brightener facial to smooth fine lines and also to promote pigment uniformity. Restore your skin's natural luster. Do it for yourself.

chapter two
Control Your Weight

28. Don't Skip Breakfast

Don't have time for it? Get up a few minutes earlier. You don't need a lot of time to prepare a nutritious breakfast. Just a small amount of healthful food can help refuel your body properly and will be worth the few minutes of lost sleep. Keep quick breakfast foods on hand, or get your breakfast foods ready the night before to save time in the morning. Avoid fast foods. While it's tempting to stop at the drive-through, these meals aren't going to do much for you in terms of health and nutrition. It's easy to stick some oatmeal with walnuts in a slow cooker at bedtime so you can have a hot treat for breakfast.

29. Snack on Almonds and Dried Cranberries or Raisins

Contrary to popular belief, snacking can be part of a healthful eating plan. Choosing snacks wisely, such as a few almonds and dried fruit, can help fuel your body between meals, give you an energy boost, and add to your total intake of essential nutrients for the day. Snacking can also help to take the edge off hunger between meals. The longer you wait between meals, the more you tend to eat at the next meal. Leaving only about three to four hours between meals is an ideal amount of time to keep blood sugar levels in control. The key to smart snacking is the type and amounts of food that you choose. Mindless snacking or nibbling on high-fat, high-calorie foods can lead to trouble in the form of unwanted and empty calories and weight gain.

30. Kick Your Exercise Session Up a Notch with Zumba

Many men and women spend big bucks on fad diets, personal trainers, dietary supplements, and other products promising a quick and easy path to weight loss. Most doctors will tell you that there's no magic formula beyond consuming fewer calories and burning more of them through exercise. If you find yoga, walking, bicycling, swimming, tennis, or golf not exciting enough to hold your interest, why not give Zumba a try? Called by some practitioners the hottest new movement in the industry of fitness, Zumba fuses Latin rhythms with easy-to-follow fast and slow movements as well as resistance training for a vigorous cardio workout. The party-style workout has broad appeal and is the brainchild of celebrity fitness expert "Beto" Perez, whose dance music tapes from his native Colombia provided the inspiration for Zumba.

31. Use Flavored Vinegars and Olive Oil in Your Salad

Salads made of fresh baby greens, a variety of lettuces, and other fresh vegetables are not only healthy but they taste good and are filling. But a pitfall of eating salad is dressings that may be high in fat, sugar, and calories. An easy way to make a tasty salad dressing is to use raspberry, pear, fig, or other fruit- or herb-flavored vinegar, and mix the vinegar with an equal amount of extra virgin olive oil. Add seasonings if you like, and put the mixture into a spray bottle to spritz on salad.

32. Restrict Your Calories to Reduce the Effects of Aging

This idea, first proposed by noted gerontologist Dr. Roy Walford of the UCLA Medical School, suggests that the effects of aging may actually be the result of too many calories over our lifetime. Through his studies, Walford concluded that a high-nutrient, low-calorie diet can have a dramatic effect in retarding the aging process by reducing weight to the point of metabolic efficiency. The downside is that the diet is very restricted. Check with your doctor before undertaking any type of diet and/or exercise regimen.

33. Toss Acai Berries into Your Cereal Bowl

This little South American berry, like other dark-skinned berries that you can wash, remove the seed, and pop fresh into your mouth as a snack or eat with your cereal, is a brain and body super food. Chock full of antioxidants and vitamins and high in protein, it also contains Omega-3s, that wonderful brain nutrient. Throw a handful into a smoothie or eat them dried or fresh. Since they come from South America, it is important that you buy only those that have been rapidly processed and preserved.

34. Use Light Tofu and Low-Sodium Soy Sauce

Chicken, shrimp, and vegetarian stir-fry dishes are easy to make, low calorie, and healthy for you. But you can further reduce the fat and cholesterol in them by choosing light tofu and low-sodium versions of soy sauce. For a simple sauce for a vegetarian stir-fry, mix together ½ cup of water, ¼ cup of sherry, 2 tablespoons soy sauce, 1 tablespoon cornstarch, 1 teaspoon sugar, and 1 table-spoon fresh chopped ginger. You can also try using a hot wok with a little water instead of oil to get your favorite vegetables steaming a bit before tossing in the tofu and stirring in the sauce. You could also add a dash of your favorite seasonings.

35. Follow the American Heart Association Dietary Guidelines

Adhere to the following eight simple guidelines for optimum health. Eat intelligently to get fit and stay fit for life. To read more, go to the American Heart Association's website at *www.americanheart. org/presenter.jhtml?identifier=532* and type into the search field the subject of your question.

- Total fat intake should be less than 25 to 30 percent of total daily calories.
- Saturated fat intake should be less than 7 percent of total daily calories.
- Trans fat should be limited to less than 1 percent of total daily calories
- Cholesterol intake should be limited to less than 300 milligrams per day.
- Choose whole-grain, high-fiber foods and a wide variety of vegetables and fruits.
- Consume at least two servings of fish twice a each week or more.
- Sodium intake should be less than 2,300 milligrams per day.

- Alcohol consumption should not exceed one drink per day for women, two for men. A drink is defined as four ounces wine, one twelve-ounce beer, one and a half ounces of 80-proof spirits, or one ounce of 100-proof spirits.

36. Try a Cup of Kombucha

Kombucha, known by the Chinese for over 2,000 years as the Immortal Health Elixir, is a fermented tea that has recently surged in popularity. Many health-conscious people use it as a supplement with nutritious food choices, while others drink the tea believing that it helps with weight control (although some sources suggest that the Tibetan Pu-erh mushroom may be more appropriate for weight loss and lower cholesterol levels). Kombucha users say the tea tastes fizzy like apple cider. The fermentation of Kombucha is accomplished via a culture that is a symbiotic, probiotic colony of yeast and bacteria. Perhaps because of the pancake shape of the culture, Kombucha also has been referred to as Kargasok mushroom and also Manchurian mushroom, although it isn't truly any type of mushroom. Before trying Kombucha tea, read the literature about it and make certain that your tea comes from a reliable source, free of contamination. Exercise caution especially if you have a depressed immune system, are pregnant, or are nursing. Be especially aware of allergic symptoms if you've never before drunk Kombucha.

37. Try a Liquid Diet for a Day

People who have gastric bypass surgery are often given a liquid diet to follow for a period of time before pureed, and then soft food is offered. If you are otherwise healthy and don't like the idea of fasting, why not try a liquid diet for a day? Focus on liquids such as broth, juices, milk, strained cream soup, water, yogurt drinks, and cooked cereal such as cream of wheat or rice. Focus on liquids that have nutritional value and stay away from high-caloric liquids with little or no nutritional value such as soda. You'll be giving your digestive track a break. And since the liquid diet is not as severe as a fast, you might find it easy and desirable to do once a week.

38. Consider Weight-Loss Surgery

If you are 100 pounds or more over your ideal weight and have tried other weight-loss therapies, treatments, and regimens with little or no weight loss, then you may be morbidly obese. The National Institutes of Health Consensus Report states that morbid obesity is a chronic disease with symptoms that have extended over a prolonged period of time. As such, it must be treated as a serious, chronic disease. A number of diseases are associated with morbid obesity, including type 2 diabetes, obesity-related heart disease, sleep apnea, infertility, high cholesterol, high blood pressure, heartburn, depression, and osteoarthritis, to name a few. Ask your doctor about bariatric surgery options and recommendations. Read about weight-loss surgery at the American Association of Bariatric Physicians, *www.asbp.org* or the American Society of Bariatric Plastic Surgeons, *www.asbps.org/aboutus.php.*

39. Trim the Fat from Your Meat

There are several ways to cut down on the amount of saturated fat in your diet. One is to make sure that all the meat you eat is as lean as possible and that all excess fat has been trimmed away before you eat it. Also, opting for turkey occasionally over pork or beef can cut the fat as well. For example, a three-ounce serving of lean, broiled turkey contains eleven grams of fat, while the same serving size of the leanest ground beef contains approximately seventeen grams of fat. Interestingly, pork, known as the other white meat, in the same proportion and also broiled, contains eighteen grams of fat. Try also replacing the saturated fat in your diet with monounsaturated fats such as olive oil, peanut oil, canola oil, and certain fish oils. This can go a long way toward reducing both your blood cholesterol levels and your risk of heart disease.

40. Eat Vegetarian Meals

Studies have linked vegetarianism with a decreased risk of obesity. The vegetarian diet contains less fat and cholesterol because vegetarians use fewer meat products (semi-vegetarian diets incorporate some fish). Besides reduced rates of obesity, vegetarians have a lower risk for developing high blood pressure and lower rates of colon cancer and diabetes. Dishes like wheat and corn wraps with tofu or chickpeas in a potato-onion curry are delicious, nutritious, and, best of all, not as fattening as the same culinary creations made with meat. Vegetarians strive to derive maximum nutrition from dishes made from vegetables, whole grains, nuts, seeds, and fruit. Find great ingredients for your vegetarian dishes at your local farmer's market or grocery stores that stock locally grown produce and choose organic whenever possible.

41. Lose That Gut Once and for All

Have you given up on ever having those "six-pack" abs you see on those television models? You may want to rethink that defeatist position because there are numerous health risks associated with belly fat. If you are a man, you are more likely than a woman to gain weight in that area, although women are not exempt. According to the Mayo Clinic staff, the medical risks associated with large bellies include heart disease, insulin resistance, stroke, type 2 diabetes, sleep apnea, high triglycerides, and low levels of the good cholesterol, high-density lipoprotein (HDL). To find out if your belly fat is inherited or if age is a factor, go to *www.mayoclinic.com/health/belly-fat/MC00054.*

42. Eat More Slowly

It takes at least twenty minutes for your stomach to signal your brain that it is full. Slowing down will help to curb the urge to go back for a second helping. It also ensures proper digestion. To slow down, between bites take sips of your beverage, put your fork down, and enjoy the conversation of others. Sit down to eat instead of eating while standing, driving, or watching television. Eating while doing other things means you are eating unconsciously and, thus, can easily consume more calories than you intended.

43. Try Raw Food

Raw food advocates say that eating food that has not been cooked has many benefits for people who want to be healthy and not heavy. The diet is based on foods that are prepared from scratch using fresh ingredients. If a particular dish needs to be served hot, then it is heated using a dehydrator that simply blows hot air that never reaches above 116°F. Practitioners claim that eating raw foods can improve skin appearance, help rid the body of unwanted pounds, and reduce the risk factors associated with heart disease (and possibly diabetes and certain types of cancer) because the diet is high in fiber and potassium and low in saturated fat and salt. Go raw if you want an energy boost. Try juicing some veggies and fruits for a quick shot of nutrition in a glass.

44. Budget the Calories You Consume

Instead of reaching for the high-fat, high-calorie foods, select those that give you the most nutrition and health benefits while offering lower calories. For example, broccoli is full of fiber, very filling, and extremely low in calories. You could eat more than three cups of broccoli and consume less than 100 calories. You wouldn't want another bite of food for a few hours. Lean meat is similar to broccoli in that an entire cup of chopped, skinless, grilled chicken breast amounts to roughly 230 calories and is a nutritious and low-calorie way to fill up! On the flip side, one bagel could cost you as much as 400 calories while providing very little nutritional value. Forget about topping it with extras like butter, cream cheese, jelly, jam, or eggs and sausage. It's a sure-fire way to pack on some pounds.

45. Keep a Food Diary

An ideal way to get into a weight-loss routine is to manage your caloric intake and become more creative with your food choices by keeping a food diary. Most people tend to drastically under-estimate the amount of calories they consume each day, which leads to confusion and frustration. If you smear jelly on your breakfast toast, write it down. If you grab a jellybean out of your coworker's candy bowl, write it down. Even your beverages count. Precisely document everything that goes into your mouth and you'll soon be able to see where you are going right, where you are going wrong, and how you should move forward. Calorie management is one way to begin taking control over your layer of belly fat.

46. Reach for Water

The brain uses 65 percent of the body's glucose, but too much or too little glucose can have a detrimental effect on brain function. When you drink a can of soda, which contains ten teaspoons of table sugar, that sugar is absorbed into a bloodstream that nor-mally only contains a total of about four teaspoons of blood sugar. The blood sugar level rockets to an excessive level, setting off alarms in the pancreas, and a large amount of insulin comes out to deal with the excess blood sugar. Some sugar is quickly ushered into the cells, including brain cells, and the rest is put into storage or into fat cells. When all this is done, maybe in about one hour, the blood sugar may fall dramatically and low blood sugar occurs. These rapid swings in blood sugar produce symptoms of impaired memory and clouded thinking. Water is important for proper hydration so make it a point to drink several glasses each day.

47. Lose 10 Percent of Your Excess Body Weight

Losing just 5 to 10 percent of excess body weight can help to reduce your risk for weight-related health problems. It lowers blood pressure, total cholesterol, low-density lipoprotein (LDL), which is bad cholesterol, triglyceride levels, and blood sugar. Lifestyle change is the healthiest and most permanent method of losing weight and decreasing the risk for serious health problems. Combining a healthy diet with increased physical activity and behavior modification is the most successful strategy for healthy weight loss and weight maintenance.

48. Make Your Body into a Fuel Guzzler

When you increase your muscle mass, you elevate your resting metabolic rate. This means that all other things being equal, your body will burn more calories even when you are doing nothing. Isn't it great to know that you will burn more calories even when you're sleeping? Studies show that for every additional pound of muscle mass, your body may burn thirty to fifty more calories per day. For example, if you work hard and gain five pounds of lean body mass from weight training, you may burn up to an additional 250 calories per day. In one week, that equals 1,750 calories. One pound is equal to 3,500 calories. So, in two weeks, after you have increased your lean body mass, if you maintain your same level of activity and food consumption as before, you could burn up to one pound of excess fat. Muscles burn energy. When it comes to calories, you want your body to be a fuel guzzler.

49. Understand That It Is Possible to Be Thin and Fat Simultaneously

A person may be small in size, yet have a very low percentage of lean body mass. It's important to remember for healthy weight management that it's not the size or shape of the body that matters; it's the relationship of lean mass to fat mass. Strength training is important to everyone, not only larger individuals, because we all need to be strong. And, it's possible to be thin and weak. Healthy bodies come in all shapes and sizes. It's important to remember that your goal to get in shape does not mean you need to become a size two or look like a cover model. Today's typical female model is 20 percent smaller than the average woman. Only 2 percent of women in America can maintain a typical model's physique without resorting to unhealthy or eating-disordered behavior.

chapter three

Eat Anti-Aging Foods

50. Eat Foods High in Omega-3 Fatty Acids

Certain fish like bluefish, herring, mackerel, rainbow trout, salmon, sardines, tuna, and whitefish are good sources of low-fat protein and are high in Omega-3 fatty acids, especially good for brain nutrition. Omega-3 essential fatty acids possess a natural anti-inflammatory known as eicosapentaenoic acid (EPA). The average American diet contains too much Omega-6 fatty acids (found in most types of vegetable oil) and too little Omega-3. If you are striving for a healthy balance, try cutting back on foods high in Omega-6 in favor of ones that are high in Omega-3.

51. Try Black Current Seed Oil

Black current seed oil, evening primrose oil, and borage oil contain the essential anti-inflammatory agent known as gamma-linolenic acid (GLA). Ingested as part of your regular diet, those oils can help strengthen your body's immune system. Black current seed oil, or *Ribes nigrum*, is particularly rich in essential fatty acids, necessary for such bodily functions as regulating body temperature, insulating nerves, providing energy, protecting tissue, and regulating metabolism. Because black current seed oil is especially high in gamma-linolenic acid, which is instrumental in making prostaglandins, it is prized as an effective anti-inflammatory herb. Prostaglandins regulate the menstrual cycle in women and black current seed oil has been used to alleviate menstrual cramping. You can usually find black current seed oil in health food stores or on the Internet. Taken in capsule form as a supplement, the recommended daily dosage is one to three 500-milligram capsules.

52. Choose Veggie Chips

To have a youthful body, you will need to give yours the right nutrition. That doesn't mean that you can eat the way you did when you were younger. Maybe you ate enough chips in your teens to take down a potato field and you never put on a pound. However, your body changes over time. Replace those salty, high-calorie chips with baked veggie chips or dried fruit snacks that are wholesome and good for you. Even better, choose to snack on crunchy raw carrots, apples, celery, broccoli, and cauliflower. What you eat profoundly affects your health, not only today, but also in your older age.

53. Eat Beans and Other Non-Meat Sources of Protein

The need for protein increases slightly as you age, yet many older people tend to eat less than they did when they were younger. In the minds of many, protein means red meat, but as you get older, it's important that you get your protein with as little fat as possible. How? Increase your consumption of fish, legumes, nuts, and grains. They can be eaten in a wide variety of ways, and they're far less expensive than meat.

54. Nibble on a Bran Muffin

A bran muffin at breakfast is a great way to start the day with a little fiber. The whole fiber phenomenon started in the 1970s, when researchers noticed that certain groups in Africa appeared to have a lower incidence of colon cancer as a result of their high fiber consumption. Later studies also found an association between high fiber intake and reduced rates of breast cancer. However, it's important to note that fiber alone may not be responsible for these benefits. Many diets high in fiber are also low in fat, and this could play an important role in reducing cancer risk. Choose low-fat bran muffins, since muffins generally contain high amounts of fat. If you make a batch at home, you can control the amount of fat and you'll have enough muffins for the whole week. Fiber is an important part of a nutritionally sound diet. Do all you can to make sure you are getting sufficient daily amounts.

55. Take Milk Thistle for Your Liver

Your liver is the only organ in your body with the ability to rejuvenate itself. It is your main source of detoxification, especially from alcohol, nicotine (including second-hand smoke), and carbon monoxide. As the liver is exposed to more and more pollutants, it has to work harder to expel them. Use of milk thistle to treat liver disease dates back two millennia. Milk thistle is indigenous to Europe's Mediterranean area as well as in the Middle East and North Africa. Almost everyone can benefit from a milk thistle diet supplement. It is primarily marketed in the United States in capsule form. Capsules containing 200 milligrams of a concentrated extract represents 140 milligrams of silymarin, a flavonoid complex found in the seeds of milk thistle. One to three tablets a day are recommended, or follow instructions on the manufacturer's label.

56. Buy Organic Foods

Increasingly, markets and groceries are stocking organic produce, fruits, beverages, and meats. Expect to pay higher prices, because it is costlier to produce items free of pesticides and raise animals for meat outside of the standard industry practices of injecting animals with hormones to fatten them before they are shipped to market or dosing them with strong antibiotics. Organic meat, for example, comes from animals that have been pasture, hay, silage, and grain fed. To be certified organic, such animals cannot have been fed any mammalian or poultry by-products. The feed mills that supply the food for organic livestock must be FDA inspected and certified. Produce, too, must meet certain criteria to be labeled organic. Make it a point to patronize organic markets, such as Whole Foods Market, North America's largest organic and natural foods retail store, The Fresh Market, with stores throughout eastern and southern United States, or health food grocery outlets in your area.

57. Check with Your Doctor Before Taking or Using Anti-Aging Products

Before taking over-the-counter anti-aging supplements or engaging in any other dramatic lifestyle or dietary changes, it's a good idea to consult with your physician if you have a chronic health condition or disability that could be affected by such changes. Certain foods can react adversely with certain medications, and some anti-aging supplements may result in physical changes that could affect medical treatment. Even though the majority of over-the-counter supplements are considered generally safe and effective, seek your doctor's approval before using such products.

58. Eat Probiotic-Rich Yogurt

You've probably seen the television ads for Activia yogurt extolling its benefits for digestive tract health. In fact, almost everyone is interested in consuming more probiotic foods because they are so healthful. Probiotic (meaning "pro life") foods introduce live organisms into the gut, whereas prebiotics are nondigestible food substances that act as food for the beneficial microorganisms that are already present in the gut. The prebiotics encourage growth and stimulate the activity of "friendly" bacteria species such as L. acidophilus and various types of bifidobacterium. There are a few preliminary studies in humans that relate the consumption of bifidobacterium to increased immunity. As it turns out, probiotic-rich yogurt is considered by many to be a superfood. In a scientific study published in the *Journal of Digestive Diseases*, individuals with some gastrointestinal disturbances benefited from eating probiotic yogurt. One study of older people indicated that a mixture of bifidobacteria and acidophilus bacteria decreased chronic inflammation of the colon and increased immunity. Existing evidence from animal and human studies suggests a moderate cholesterol-lowering action of fermented dairy products. If you suffer from irregularity or gastrointestinal discomfort, give probiotics a try. Put a cup of plain, unflavored yogurt into a blender and purée it with steamed broccoli for a healthy soup or vegetable dip, or put strawberries, raspberries, or bananas in the yogurt and blend into a smoothie.

59. Develop a Taste for Sushi and Seaweed

The oceans provide an amazing quantity of mineral-rich foods that rival the most nutrient-dense land produce. Of these, dulse, arame, hijiki, and kombu are proving themselves to be effective in weight-loss studies and preventing osteoporosis. A favorite first course in Japanese restaurants is miso soup. It contains dried seaweed and tofu, tastes delicious, and is easy to make using the following recipe. Serves 4.

5 cups vegetable or mushroom stock
1 piece kombu (kelp, a dried seaweed), about 5 inches square
1 teaspoon soy sauce
3 tablespoons light (yellow) miso, such as shiro mugi miso
2 scallions, chopped
2 ounces firm tofu, diced into small cubes
4 teaspoons wakame seaweed (instant)

1. Bring stock and kombu to a boil in a soup pot. Cover; remove from heat and let stand 5 minutes. Strain; stir in soy sauce.
2. In a mixing bowl, mix about ¼ cup of the warm stock into the miso paste with a wire whisk until the miso is dissolved. Pour this mixture back into the remaining stock. Place scallions, diced tofu, and wakame into four bowls. Gently ladle soup into the bowls.

60. Enjoy an Avocado

Indigenous to Mexico, the avocado is called "aguacate" in Spanish. Avocado is a superfood because it is highly nutritious, containing vitamin K, B6, and C as well as potassium, folic acid, and copper. Also known as the butter pear, a single medium-sized avocado can contain 30 grams of fat, as much as a quarter-pound burger. But most of the fat is monounsaturated and because avocados contain oleic acid, a monounsaturated fat believed beneficial for lowering cholesterol, eating an avocado a day might not be a bad idea. A 1996 Mexican scientific study on forty-five people who ate an avocado daily for a week showed surprising health benefits: Blood cholesterol of the subjects in the study dropped an average of 17 percent, triglycerides and LDL (unhealthy fat) decreased, and HDL (which tends to reduce the risk of heart disease) increased. Besides eating the fruit cut into slices or cubes, you can scoop it out of the shell, throw away the seed, and then mash the avocado onto a small plate. Replace the cream cheese or butter on bagels and muffins and forgo the mayonnaise on your sandwich and, instead, spread on mashed avocado.

61. Snack on Pumpkin Seeds

Pumpkin seeds are one of those nutrient-rich superfoods that you want to have more of in your diet. With the slow deterioration of our food supply due to poor-quality soil, use of toxic pesticides and herbicides, genetic engineering of plants, and a host of chemicals used to preserve, color and flavor, and stimulate and addict your senses; coming back to the essential basics of whole foods is a good move. Superfoods provide essential vitamins, minerals, trace minerals, phytonutrients, antioxidants, proteins, carbohydrates, and good fats necessary to help meet your daily nutritional needs, and they are delicious to eat as well. Pumpkin seeds are high in minerals, proteins, and phytosterols, believed to reduced levels of LDL. Toast them in the oven with a little sea salt for a tasty snack.

62. Learn about Macronutrients and Micronutrients

Most foods contain a combination of two groups that you will want to include when planning your food menu: *macronutrients*, so called because the body needs more of them; and *micronutrients*, nutrients required in only small amounts—these include vitamins and minerals. Macronutrients include carbohydrates, fats, and proteins, which are the foods your body uses for energy and growth. Both are necessary for good health and a strong immune system if you want to feel good and look your best. When planning your menu or snack, try to include each of the macronutrients to ensure well-balanced meals.

63. Drink a Glass of Wine a Day

One glass of wine for women and two for men has been proven to reduce the risk of certain cancers and heart disease as well as slowing the progression of Alzheimer's and Parkinson's disease, according to some research. However, the health benefit is forfeited if you drink more than that. Wine has non-alcoholic phytochemicals (flavanoids and resveratol) that prevent free radical molecules from damaging your body's cells. A glass a day will do more good than harm, so enjoy that glass with dinner.

64. Eat Quinoa

If you haven't heard of this ancient grain, once considered sacred by the Incas, ask for it at your local health food store or at a Whole Foods market. Cooked quinoa (pronounced KEEN-wah) is chewy with a nutty taste. It has grown for more than 5,000 years in the Andes, and the ancient Incas considered it the mother of all grains. However, it isn't truly a grain but rather a seed from a Peruvian plant (chenopodium quinoa) that is related to beets, spinach, and also chard. It contains all nine of the essential amino acids and, therefore, is a complete protein. It also contains copper, phosphorus, and manganese as well as magnesium. Because of its high protein content and nutrient value, the United Nations classified it a superfood. Rinse the seeds in cold water and prepare as a hot cereal (add some fresh or dried fruit and honey) or in your favorite soup.

65. Reject the Steak and Order the Fish

Fish is a better choice for a meal than a heavily marbled steak, especially if it comes with a giant helping of fries, mashed potatoes, or potatoes au gratin (with cheese). Depending on how it is prepared, the fish will be lower in calories and cholesterol than the steak (not to mention the calories and fat in those potatoes because of how they are prepared); a boon for your waistline and your overall health. Some fish oils and types of fish, such as bluefish, herring, mackerel, rainbow trout, salmon, sardines, tuna, and whitefish are high in omega-3 fatty acids (important for brain nutrition).

66. Eat Fish Low in Mercury Content

Fish is high in omega-3 oils, so it's very healthy, but some fish has a higher mercury content. The FDA and EPA recommends limited consumption of shark, swordfish, king mackerel, or tilefish because they contain high levels of mercury. They also recommend no more than six ounces (170 grams) per week of canned albacore ("white") tuna, tuna steaks, lobster, halibut, and orange roughy. A six-ounce serving is about the size of two decks of cards or two checkbooks. The FDA also recommends that you eat no more than twelve ounces (340 grams) per week of fish and shellfish lower in mercury. This equates to two average six-ounce (170-gram) meals. Fish lower in mercury include canned light tuna (not albacore tuna), salmon, pollock, catfish, cod, crab, flounder/sole, grouper, haddock, herring, mahi-mahi, ocean perch, oysters, sardines, scallops, shrimp, tilapia, and trout.

67. Know Your Fibers

There are four major types of fiber, each of which can benefit your body in a special way:

- **Cellulose.** This is the most common type of fiber and is found in most fruits and vegetables, as well as whole grains and some types of nuts. Cellulose is an effective stool softener and helps dilute bile acids in the colon, which are believed to stimulate the growth of certain types of cancer.
- **Gums.** These are sticky fibers derived from plants. They help lower cholesterol and prevent certain types of cancer, though researchers are still trying to figure out exactly how they work. Gums are found in oat bran, dried beans, and oatmeal and are commonly used to thicken processed foods.
- **Lignin.** This fiber acts as a binder for cellulose and is found in certain fruits, nuts, peas, tomatoes, and whole grains. It doesn't have the same action as cellulose on stools or bile acids, but laboratory studies have shown that it can help prevent the onset of cancer.
- **Pectin.** This gelatinous compound supplements the action of cellulose. It helps limit the potential damage from bile acids and also aids digestion by preventing diarrhea. Rich sources of pectin include apples, bananas, beets, carrots, and a wide array of citrus fruit.

68. Consume Dairy Products for Calcium, but Stick to Low Fat

Dairy products are a good source of calcium as well as other vitamins and minerals, but they should be low fat if possible. People who are lactose intolerant should explore nondairy alternatives and should consider taking calcium supplements to prevent age-related osteoporosis and similar disorders. Non-lactose-intolerant people can get calcium in dairy products including milk, ice cream, pudding, yogurt, and cheese, for example. Also, nondairy soy products such as tofu and fortified soy drinks contain calcium as well as protein.

69. Limit Trans Fat in Your Diet

Another name for trans fat (trans fatty acids) is "partially hydrogenated vegetable oils." Eating trans fat raises levels of your LDL or "bad" cholesterol and lowers levels of your HDL or "good" cholesterol. Eating trans fat is associated with higher risk of stroke and heart disease, and also for developing diabetes. Limiting or excluding trans fat in your diet can reduce your risks. Make it a habit to search ingredient listings on packages and in food products for trans fats or partially hydrogenated vegetable oils. Avoid foods that are known to contain trans fat such as fried foods (for example French fries and doughnuts) and many baked goods like pies, cakes, cookies, crackers, stick margarines and fats. Choose foods instead that are made with monounsaturated or polyunsaturated fats.

chapter four

Repel Heart Disease and Cancer

70. Eat Dark Chocolate for Heart Health

Dark chocolate may help lower blood pressure in people with hypertension, and has been shown to decrease levels of LDL, the "bad" cholesterol, by 10 percent. Including dark chocolate in your diet may benefit your heart by helping to block arterial damage caused by free radicals, and inhibit platelet aggregation, which could cause a heart attack or stroke. There have also been studies indicating that the flavonoids in cocoa relax the blood vessels, which inhibits an enzyme that causes inflammation.

71. Put Away the Salt Shaker

Reduce your intake of sodium. It is important to have a proper balance of both potassium and sodium in the diet but many people get enough sodium every day and still add salt to almost everything, including sweet melon. Most guidelines suggest that adults consume no more than 2,300 milligrams. daily of salt. That's the equivalent of one teaspoon. Check food labels for listings of amounts of sodium contained in the product. You'll see that sodium is in almost everything. Avoid processed foods, which are often high in sodium. Instead of using salt to season food, try a variety of herbs and spices.

72. Increase Potassium Consumption

Potassium is an electrolyte that works closely with its counterparts, chloride and sodium. Over 95 percent of potassium is in the body's cells and helps regulate the flow of fluids and minerals in and out of the body's cells. It also helps maintain normal blood pressure, maintain heart and kidney function, and transmit nerve impulses and contraction of muscles. Studies have also shown that potassium may also reduce the risk of high blood pressure and stroke. Potassium is widely available in baked sweet potatoes (containing the highest levels of potassium) as well as beet greens, baked potatoes, white beans, clams, carrot juice, plain low-fat yogurt, prune juice, lima beans, winter squash, and bananas, to name a few food sources Most people excrete excess potassium in their urine. If the excess cannot be excreted (by someone with kidney disease, for example), it can cause heart problems. Some experts recommend a higher intake, around 3,500 milligrams per day, to help protect against high blood pressure, but check with your doctor first.

73. Balance Potassium and Sodium Levels in Your Diet

It is important to have a proper balance of both potassium and sodium in the diet. Studies have indicated a possible link between a diet high in sodium and low in potassium and an increased risk of cancer, heart disease, high blood pressure, and stroke. On the other hand, a diet high in potassium and low in sodium may help to protect or decrease the risk for these health problems. Stay vigilant about what you eat. Read labels and check the levels of sodium and potassium listed. Some canned soups, for example, a common meal for many people on the go, can contain high levels of sodium and are generally taboo for someone on a low-sodium diet.

74. Take Heart-Healthy Herbs to Curb Stress

Chronic stress can cause your brain to release cortisol, the powerful hormone that regulates the "fight or flight" response. Cortisol, in elevated levels, is bad for your heart and can also negatively impact your sleep, mood, and libido. If you have a lot of daily stress, check with your doctor about trying some herbs that calm anxiety and tension. Specifically, you might consider pasque flower, also known as the Easter flower and May Day flower because of the timing of its appearance in the spring. Scullcap, wood betony, and vervain also have properties that can relieve stress. Scullcap acts as a relaxant and restorative for the central nervous system and is beneficial for nervous debility. Wood betony is a sedative that acts to calm the nervous system by soothing fearfulness and invigorating exhaustion. Finally, vervain calms nerves and has a tonic effect on the liver.

75. Drink Hawthorn Tea

Does your family have a history of heart disease? Ask your doctor if you can use hawthorn. The herb has been scientifically proven to lower high blood pressure, promote overall improvement in heart health and blood flow, ease angina and shortness of breath, reduce swollen ankles, and improve strength and circulation in people with congestive heart failure. Hawthorn contains rutin, a substance that reduces the formation and buildup of plaque, which can block blood flow and possibly lead to stroke or a heart attack. Finally, the herb is effective against arrhythmia, heart rhythm disturbances.

Take one 300-milligram tablet per day, or one tablespoon of dried berries in one cup of boiling water, steeped for ten minutes.

76. Eat Your Oatmeal to Lower Your Cholesterol

Studies have shown that foods that are high in soluble fiber such as oat bran may help to lower LDL (bad cholesterol) without lowering HDL (good cholesterol). Whether you choose steel-cut oats (the least processed), rolled or "old-fashioned" oats, quick oats, or instant, all types of oats are effective at reducing cholesterol. The effective soluble fiber in oats (and also in barley), called beta-glucan, forms a gel that traps bile acids, which contain a lot of cholesterol, and carries them out of the body. In response, your liver makes more bile acids, which requires it to take more cholesterol out of your blood. Get three grams of soluble fiber daily for the cholesterol-lowering benefit: two cups cooked oatmeal or one and a half cups cooked oat bran. Excess cholesterol in the blood can clog arteries and lead to heart attack and stroke.

77. Consider Antidepressants to Repel a Future Cardiac Event

If you've already experienced one heart attack, antidepressants may hold the key to avoiding another one. According to Stanford University researchers conducting a study of 1,800 depressed and socially isolated individuals who had experienced at least one heart attack, psychotherapy alone was not enough to repel a second cardiac event. But taking antidepressants did reduce the risk of suffering another heart attack. The study was designed to evaluate the use of psychotherapy in patients who had previously experienced a heart event. However, antidepressants were prescribed for those patients whose depression did not respond to the cognitive behavioral therapy. The findings showed that use of the antidepressant was associated with a 43 percent lower risk of death and also a 43 percent lower risk of a future nonfatal heart attack.

78. Eat Salads with Garlic, Chives, Scallions, and Onions

Research published in the Journal of the National Cancer Institute in 2002 presented an interesting case for the reduction of men's prostate cancer risk through a diet rich in garlic and onions. After examining men's diets (238 men with prostate cancer and 471 without), researchers discovered that the men who ate more than one-third ounce of onions, garlic, chives, or scallions daily were less likely to be in the group that had cancer. Science has also linked eating allium vegetables (onions, garlic, shallots, leeks, and chives) to a decreased risk of cancers of the stomach, colon, and esophagus. Women might want to add chives, onions, and garlic to their salads, too, since there is also a lower risk associated between those foods and breast and uterine-lining cancers. See *http://jnci.oxfordjournals.org/cgi/content/abstract/94/21/1648*.

79. Protect Against Heart Disease

Consume at least twenty-five to thirty grams of fiber each day from sources such as whole grains, fruits, vegetables, and legumes. Consuming a variety of fruits and vegetables will also ensure that you receive plenty of beta-carotene, vitamin C, folic acid, vitamin E, and other antioxidants and protective substances such as flavonoids and carotenoids. You can regularly add foods such as soy, oat bran, fish, nuts, seeds, and garlic to strengthen your disease-fighting prevention diet even more. Talk to your doctor about your risk for heart disease and how to manage any risk factors you may have.

80. Eat Soyburgers

According to experts, soy protein appears to help prevent heart disease by lowering blood cholesterol levels; decreasing blood clots and platelet "clumping" or aggregation (both of which can increase the risk for a heart attack or stroke); improving the elasticity of arteries (which makes blood flow better); and reducing oxidation of LDL (bad cholesterol), which can lower the risk of plaque formation. The Food and Drug Administration is so convinced of soy's benefits that the agency approved a health claim for soy protein and heart disease in October 1999. Good sources include defattened soy flour, isolated soy protein, miso, firm tofu, regular tofu, soy cheese, soymilk, and soy veggie burgers. Adding one serving a day can make a difference. Soy up!

81. Consume Isoflavone-Rich Foods—Peas, Beans, Lentils, and Soy

What are isoflavones? They belong to a group of compounds called phytoestrogens—plant compounds that act like the human hormone estrogen in the body. Isoflavones are found in a number of plants but only soybeans provide a significant amount of phytoestrogens. These are believed to possibly reduce the risk of breast cancer and other estrogen-dependent cancers, increase bone mineral density, and reduce bone loss at the spine as well as diminish symptoms associated with menopause such as hot flashes, night sweats, vaginal dryness, and mood swings. A study examining the effect of legumes on cardiovascular health followed men and women for nineteen years. In that study those who consumed dry beans, peas, or peanuts four times weekly reduced their risk of cardiovascular disease by 21 percent over those individuals who ate those foods less than once weekly. See *http://lpi.oregonstate.edu/infocenter/foods/legumes/#intro.*

82. Take Coenzyme Q10

Coenzyme Q10 (CoQ10), also called ubiquinone, is a naturally occurring compound found in plants and animals. Levels are believed to decrease as you get older and also in people who suffer from chronic disease. The Mayo Clinic notes that some prescription drugs also may lower CoQ10. It is usually taken by mouth—tablet or capsule—but also may be administered by injection into a vein. Coenzyme Q10 is necessary for mitochondria—the energy-generating components of all cells—to work properly. Because mitochondria are found in great abundance in the cells of heart tissue, much research has been focused on CoQ10 and heart disease. For instance, CoQ10 has been shown to be useful in abnormalities involving the heart's ability to contract and pump blood effectively, such as congestive heart failure, and a number of cardiomyopathies (heart muscle diseases). Also, CoQ10 is a potent antioxidant and, as such, appears to protect vitamin E, which helps prevent the oxidation of LDL. Coenzyme Q10 may reduce the ability of blood to clot and also shows promise in helping patients with hypertension, heart valve replacement, and angina. Talk with your doctor about supplementing with CoQ10.

83. Forgo the Fish Oil Supplements for the Real Thing

An Italian study spanning thirteen years revealed that people who ate fish once weekly had a 20 to 30 percent lower risk of cancers of the mouth, stomach, esophagus, pancreas, colon, and rectum than those who ate less than one serving of fish per week. For people consuming two or more servings of fish per week, the risk dropped even lower. The researchers suggest that the protective effect of the fish may be due to its omega-3 fatty acid content believed to play an important role in the prevention and treatment of cancer. The best way to get your omega-3s is by eating salmon, herring, sardines, halibut, tuna, mackerel, and anchovies. Forgo the fish oil supplements because the production of fish oil supplements is not well regulated and some may contain heavy metals (such as mercury), pesticides, and PCBs.

84. Take Psyllium to Protect Against Heart Disease

Approximately 52 million Americans have elevated cholesterol levels. If you are one of them, you should know that psyllium, a soluble fiber—the "sticky" form that thickens the contents of the intestines and slows the digestion/absorption process—appears to play a protective role against diabetes and heart disease. For many years, psyllium has been recommended as a means to increase fecal bulk and loosen stools. As a source of water-soluble fiber, the psyllium husk (which contains small seeds) is similar to barley and oat bran. It is much higher in fiber, however, than oat bran. More recently, studies have shown that psyllium intake seems to decrease blood cholesterol levels, a risk factor in cardiovascular disease. A number of studies have reported a significant decline in death due to coronary heart disease (CHD) as a result of lowering blood cholesterol levels. Of the fifty-five studies done over the last thirty years that linked psyllium intake to blood cholesterol, only three did not show a reduction in cholesterol levels. The Food and Drug Administration recently granted a health claim for psyllium. Take psyllium as a powder, whole husks (stirred into soups or smoothies), or in capsule form. Drink at least one full eight-ounce glass of water or juice after taking a psyllium capsule. If you want to use psyllium in your weight-loss effort, take it with a glass of liquid at least thirty minutes before a meal. The full feeling will help curb your appetite.

85. Increase Beta-Carotene in Your Diet

Beta-carotene is found in a variety of fruits and vegetables, especially those that are bright yellow or orange, and dark, leafy greens. Interestingly, beta-carotene absorption is much better from cooked produce than from raw. Steaming vegetables will increase the availability of beta-carotene, although overcooking can destroy this carotenoid. Because the carotenoids are fat soluble, eating beta-carotene with a little fat or oil will also increase absorption. A large body of evidence suggests that high blood levels of carotenoids may reduce the risk of cancer, heart disease, cataracts, and macular degeneration, the leading cause of irreversible blindness in old age.

86. Know the Heart-Health Risks of Sleep Apnea

Ninety percent of the people who suffer from sleep apnea (a disruption of sleep that has serious cardiovascular ramifications) don't even know they have it. Symptoms of sleep apnea include: choking or gasping for air, frequent and sometimes prolonged silences, loud snoring, and drowsiness during the day, possibly even falling asleep at inappropriate times. People with sleep apnea have a higher risk for developing cardiovascular disease. New research suggests that even people who suffer from mild sleep apnea have cause for concern. Scientists studied the artery stiffness as well as the functioning of the endothelial cells lining the blood vessels in sixty-four patients with mild sleep apnea and fifteen individuals without sleep apnea. They found decreased endothelial function and greater artery stiffness in patients with sleep apnea. A similar study on those two groups of blood pressure revealed similar findings, indicating that serious, even life-threatening health consequences are associated with sleep apnea. Some of the things you can do to alleviate sleep apnea include losing weight, stopping drinking and smoking, elevating your head to help stop snoring, sleeping on your side, avoiding sedatives, and using aids to open nasal passages (such as breathing strips and saline nasal spray). Consult with your doctor if you have sleep apnea symptoms.

87. Take Iron to Prevent Iron-Deficiency Anemia

Iron creates healthy red blood cells that can carry oxygen to all of your body's tissues, creating energy, and giving a healthy glow to your skin. The U.S. Food and Drug Administration recommends that women who are in their childbearing years and who may become pregnant should consume foods rich in heme-iron (easily absorbed iron from meat), eat plant foods that are iron-rich, and/ or eat iron-fortified foods with an iron-absorption enhancer (for example, foods with high amounts of vitamin C). A common health issue for close to 18 million Americans is iron-deficiency anemia, a condition that occurs when blood lacks the proper amount of iron. Iron-deficiency anemia is most often found in women, with symptoms ranging from pale skin to commonly feeling fatigued. Anemia can also cause headaches, stomach disorders, restless-leg syndrome, and a loss of libido. Not supplementing your diet with iron-rich foods can increase your risk of developing anemia, but a daily serving of quinoa, with 2.8 milligrams of iron per one-cup serving, can alleviate worries about getting enough iron.

88. Add Red Fruits and Veggies High in Lycopene to Your Diet

Lycopene (pronounced LIE-co-peen) is a carotenoid, or natural pigment, that gives tomatoes and watermelon their deep red color. It is the predominant carotenoid in the body—found in human blood and tissue—but it's derived entirely from food sources. Lycopene is also a powerful antioxidant and phytochemical. Studies show that phytochemicals (naturally occurring chemical components found in fruits, vegetables, legumes, and grains) may reduce the incidence and severity of certain diseases. For instance, a growing body of research suggests that lycopene may help reduce the risk of heart disease and some cancers. In a recent study, men with prostate cancer who took thirty milligrams of lycopene per day (equal to about a half cup of spaghetti sauce), for three weeks, had a reduction in tumor size and malignancy.

89. Develop a Taste for Onions

You may not like onions, but if researchers at the German Institute of Human Nutrition in Potsdam-Rehbruecke along with their colleagues from California and Hawaii are right, the lowly onion may, in fact, be effective in repelling pancreatic cancer. The study involved more than 215,000 subjects in California and Hawaii over a three-year period from 1996 to 1999. From the participants' dietary information, scientists were able to assess the association between flavonols (found in a variety of fruits and vegetables and believed to have cancer-fighting properties) and risk of cancer. Although more research is needed, the findings indicate that a higher total intake of flavonols was associated with lower risk of pancreatic cancer. Three flavonols in the study included kaempferol (abundant in spinach and certain cabbages), quercetin (found in onions and apples), and myricetin (contained in red onions and berries).

90. Make a Donation to Fight Cancer

You might wonder how this could help you look and feel younger, but just imagine how disfiguring skin cancer is on the face. If cancer is not on the face but in an ovary, the prostate, or the breast, it may not only be disfiguring but life threatening. If a cure is found for any of the various types of cancer, the discovery might save your life should you ever be stricken with some form of that terrible disease. Show your support for the fight against cancer. Donate to the Livestrong campaign and wear its yellow wristband. This organization was started by Lance Armstrong and holds bike races all around the country to raise money. Go to *www.livestrong.org* to learn more and make your donation.

chapter five

Supplement with Vitamins and Minerals

91. Take Daily Supplements for Nutritional Gaps

Dr. Andrew Weil, director of the integrative medicine program at the University of Arizona in Tucson, advised viewers of television's *Good Morning America* that they should consider taking a comprehensive antioxidant and multivitamin regimen if they were concerned about nutritional gaps in their daily diet. His specific recommendation included 200 milligrams of vitamin C, 400 to 800 IU of natural vitamin E (or 80 milligrams of mixed tocopherols and tocotrienols), 200 micrograms of selenium, 15,000 to 20,000 IU of mixed carotenoids, and 30 to 100 milligrams of coenzyme Q10. Vitamins, from both food and supplements, are necessary for the growth of cells, to help your bodily systems function properly, and provide energy and vitality.

92. Compare Vitamin Supplement Prices and Potency Levels

Store-brand supplements—especially those from larger chains—are often the best bargain and are equal in quality to the higher-priced supplements advertised on television or available from specialty outlets. The least you can expect to pay for a multivitamin and mineral supplement is $1 to $5 for a one-month supply (one tablet per day). When comparing prices online, be sure to factor in shipping and handling charges. Check that the supplement manufacturer uses Good Manufacturing Practices (GMPs) before purchasing their products. Good Manufacturing Practices ensure that the product and the potency level match what's indicated on the label. If the label has the seal of the National Nutritional Foods

Association, it means that the manufacturer meets the association's standards for quality.

93. Understand the Way Water-Soluble Vitamins Work

High concentrations of water-soluble vitamins travel freely throughout the bloodstream. The kidneys are sensitive to high concentrations of substances in the blood. When particular substances are in excess, the kidneys remove them and pass them into the urine. This includes the water-soluble vitamins—high doses of most of these vitamins are simply passed into the urine.

94. Gain the Health Benefits of Vitamin B6

Vitamin B6 supplementation has been used in the treatment of, or in an attempt to prevent, a number of diseases, including Down syndrome, autism, gestational diabetes (diabetes during pregnancy), premenstrual syndrome, CTS, and diabetic neuropathy. However, B6 supplementation has been of limited benefit in those circumstances. And in some cases, such as the treatment of premenstrual syndrome, supplementing with B6 has resulted in a small number of cases of neurotoxicity (which can cause a loss of sensation in hands and feet and an inability to walk) and photosensitivity. These symptoms are usually seen when doses above 500 milligrams per day are used. Additionally, findings from the Nurses' Health Study showed that women with the highest intakes of vitamin B6 and folate had a lower risk of coronary heart disease than women with lower intakes of these vitamins. Eat foods high in vitamin B6 such as liver, bananas, chicken, pistachios, halibut, pork chops, and prunes, to name a few.

95. Take Folic Acid in Synthetic Form

Folic acid is one of those nutrients better absorbed in the synthetic, or man-made, form than it is from food. Folate, the version of the B vitamin found in food, is absorbed by the body half as well as folic acid, which is the form found in fortified foods and supplements. In the case of vitamin B12, up to one-third of people over the age of fifty have trouble absorbing this vitamin from food. Therefore, the National Academy of Sciences recommends that people in these age groups obtain both of these nutrients from fortified foods and/or supplements. Folic acid is a must for women of childbearing age. Get it either through fortified foods or a supplement—most multivitamins contain the recommended 400 micrograms.

96. Know the Health Risks of Fat-Soluble Vitamins

Vitamins A, D, E, and K in small amounts are important for maintaining excellent health. Bile acids (fluids your body uses to absorb fat) act to absorb and store these vitamins until needed. You gain health benefits consuming foods rich in those vitamins and the body does not require daily intake of them. These vitamins are not as easily excreted from the body as the water-soluble vitamins. Health problems can occur, however, if these four vitamins are taken in mega doses because in high doses, they can be toxic.

97. Reach for a Liquid Nutritional Supplement

As you age, your nutritional needs change. So does your attitude toward nutrition and food. You might have a diminished appetite because of medications you have to take, your activity level has dropped, and your metabolism has slowed. You might have started skipping meals because of fatigue or lack of interest, are battling a debilitating illness, or are recovering from an operation. Whatever the reason, if you suspect you aren't getting adequate nutrition, try a liquid supplement chocked full of the nutrients your body needs, including the proper balance of vitamins, minerals, protein, antioxidants, fiber, calcium, and carbohydrates. Many are formulated to meet special nutritional needs. Numerous scientific studies have shown that nutritional drinks like Boost, Ensure, Sustacal, and Glucerna (formulated for diabetics) are good sources of supplemental nutrition and offer health benefits to seniors including mood elevation, better cognition, and increased energy.

98. Understand Vitamin C's Possible Protection Against Cataracts

Researchers at Tufts and Harvard Universities studied nearly 250 women with no history of cataracts. Those who had been supplementing with vitamin C for at least ten years had 77 percent fewer early-stage opacities (the first sign of cataracts) and 83 percent fewer moderate opacities than women who did not supplement. Although there is much debate among the experts regarding how much vitamin C is necessary for this protective effect, 150 to 200 milligrams is the amount needed to saturate eye tissues.

99. Know the Signs of Vitamin D Deficiency

Surveys indicate that the usual dietary intake of vitamin D in the United States is low—50 to 70 IU per day. Presumably, vitamin D stores are enriched in most people by regular exposure to sunlight, at least during certain times of the year. Recommended intake for vitamin D for males and females aged fifty-one to seventy is 400 IU, or 600 IU per day if over age seventy. Rickets is perhaps the best-known classic example of vitamin D deficiency. It is characterized by the bowing of long bones (in children, bones that are still developing) because of impaired mineralization due to lack of vitamin D in the diet and also lack of exposure to sunlight. The symptoms of vitamin D deficiency include muscle twitching, cramps, and convulsions, as well as aching bones. Adults who are vitamin D deficient develop osteomalacia. The disease doesn't cause bone deformities, but it does result in a decrease of the mineral content of the bones, leaving them more prone to fractures.

100. Take an Extra Dose of Vitamin D

Among the nutritional tips put out by the School of Public Health at Harvard is the suggestion that extra vitamin D might offer a health boost because that vitamin lowers the risk of colon cancer and possibly several other cancers as well. See *www.hsph .harvard.edu/nutritionsource/what-should-you-eat/vitamins*. And a paper published by the University of Colorado states that vitamin D has potent physiological effects broader than just bone function. In fact, many (if not most) of the cells in the human body have vitamin D receptors. Read more at *www.vivo.colostate.edu/ hbooks/pathphys/endocrine/otherendo/vitamind.html*. In a University of Manchester study involving 3,000 men, ages forty to seventy-nine, the scientists compared the test subjects' cognitive performances and found that middle-aged men who had higher levels of vitamin D from sunlight exposure and certain foods performed the best on cognitive function tests, whereas lower levels of vitamin D in older men showed an association with decreased cognitive function. NaturalNews.com has also reported that vitamin D from exposure to sunlight and through diet may reduce the risk of breast cancer tumors. Read more at *www.naturalnews .com/025495.html.*

101. Consider Daily Doses of Vitamin E

A number of epidemiological studies suggest that low blood levels or intakes of vitamin E are associated with increased risk of certain types of cancer. Occurrence of cancer of the stomach, esophagus, and cervix seems to be reduced when antioxidant supplements (including vitamin E) are taken for a period of years. Vitamin E supplements have also been associated with lower risk of oral, colon, breast, thyroid, prostate, gastrointestinal tract, lung, and bladder cancers. In many cases, at least 100 IU of vitamin E per day is needed. In a two-year study of people with Alzheimer's disease, progression of the disease was slowed when either 2,000 IU of vitamin E (alpha-tocopherol), 10 milligrams of Selegiline, or a combination of the two was taken daily.

102. Take Vitamin C to Reduce Symptoms of Exercise-Induced Asthma

Vitamin C may help people with exercise-induced asthma (EIA) breathe more easily. In a well-controlled study from Israel, individuals with EIA were given a single dose of 2,000 milligrams of vitamin C one hour before exercising on a treadmill. The researchers found that ascorbic acid prevented or decreased the severity of wheezing attacks and lung discomfort in over half of the study participants. It appears that vitamin C may protect against damaging oxidants in the lungs.

103. Consider the Importance of Vitamin K

Vitamin K is best known for its important role in blood clotting. At least thirteen different proteins are involved in making a blood clot, and vitamin K is essential for the production of at least six of them—especially the protein thrombin. If any of these important proteins are missing, blood cannot clot, which results in hemorrhagic disease. In other words, if an artery or vein is cut, the bleeding will not stop. Hemorrhagic disease is caused by a vitamin K deficiency, which can occur as a result of fat malabsorption (from liver disease, Crohn's disease, or ulcerative colitis) or destruction of the intestinal bacteria by prolonged use of antibiotics. Prior to surgery, patients sometimes are given vitamin K to prevent excess bleeding during an operation, but only if a known vitamin K deficiency exists. Until recently, researchers believed that the body made all of the vitamin K it needed. But new studies indicate that even though the body may make enough vitamin K for blood clotting, it's not necessarily enough for good bone health. In fact, the current RDAs for vitamin K may be too low.

104. Take Note of Chromium's Health Benefits

Chromium, a mineral that helps the body metabolize fat, convert blood sugar into energy, and make insulin work more efficiently, is derived primarily from diets rich in whole-grain foods, eggs, broccoli, orange juice, grape juice, seafood, dairy products, and many different types of meat. Chromium is also available in supplement form. Studies have also shown that chromium protects the heart by lowering serum cholesterol levels and triglycerides. It also seems to prevent or aid in the management of diabetes by assisting in the production and metabolism of insulin. Additionally, it increases muscle mass (with exercise), and it boosts longevity (at least in studies using laboratory rats).

105. Ward off Gallbladder Disease with Vitamin C

A recent study indicates that women who don't get enough vitamin C may be at a greater risk for gallbladder disease. Gallstones are often formed when bile, a liquid formed by the liver to help break down fats during digestion, becomes saturated with cholesterol. Vitamin C helps break down cholesterol, preventing it from hardening into gallstones, which can grow up to one inch across and cause severe abdominal pain. In some cases, the gallbladder must be surgically removed. Gallstones affect many more women than men. This may be due, in part, to the fact that estrogen increases the concentration of cholesterol in bile—and most gallstones are made up of cholesterol. The findings from this latest study indicate that women who have higher blood levels of vitamin C and those who take vitamin C supplements have a lower risk of gallstones and gallbladder disease.

106. Understand How Magnesium Maintains Youthfulness

Magnesium is an important mineral that shows great promise as an anti-aging facilitator. It plays a wide variety of roles within the body but is best known for promoting the absorption and use of other minerals, including calcium. Magnesium also helps move sodium and potassium across the cell membranes, aids in the metabolism of proteins, and activates a variety of important enzymes. Taking magnesium is important for maintaining strong bones and teeth, a healthy nervous system, a balanced metabolism, and well-functioning muscles—including the heart. As far back as the 1950s, animal studies proved that high doses of magnesium can effectively reverse atherosclerotic plaques and improve blood flow to the heart. There is also strong evidence that magnesium can facilitate glucose metabolism, lowering the risk of developing diabetes and making the condition easier to manage among those who already have it.

107. Keep That Anti-Aging Selenium at a Sufficient Level

Selenium levels tend to drop precipitously as we age, which is why it's important that we maintain sufficient levels in our later years. Since the 1950s, numerous studies have placed selenium in the forefront of anti-aging research because of its suspected ability to prevent a variety of life-threatening conditions, including cancer and heart disease. Selenium is an antioxidant, working with glutathione peroxidase to keep potentially damaging free radicals under control. It also plays a role in the metabolism of prostaglandins, important hormone-like compounds that affect several essential body functions. Natural sources of selenium include broccoli, cabbage, celery, cucumbers, garlic, onions, kidney, liver, chicken, whole-grain foods, seafood, and milk. It is also available in supplement form.

108. Take Chondroitin to Improve Joint Function

Osteoarthritis occurs when the cartilage that cushions the ends of bone joints breaks down, resulting in stiff joints, joint pain, and deformity. There have been several human studies that suggest chondroitin is an effective treatment for osteoarthritis. In one study of 119 people, those who took 1,200 milligrams of chondroitin sulfate showed reduced rates of severe joint damage: only 8.8 percent of them developed severely damaged joints during the study, compared to 30 percent of those in the placebo group. And, in many of the studies, those subjects who received chondroitin rated their arthritis improvement and pain relief higher than those receiving either a prescription pain reliever or a placebo. Chondroitin is thought to give cartilage elasticity, which may improve joint function. It may also block enzymes that break down cartilage, thereby slowing the progression of osteoarthritis. Chondroitin may also increase the amount of lubricating fluid in the joints and have a mild anti-inflammatory effect.

109. Boost Your HDL (Good) Cholesterol with Niacin Supplements

A lot of media attention is focused on ways to lower LDL (bad) cholesterol levels, but raising the HDL (good) cholesterol also should be an important goal for almost everyone. A Mayo Clinic report stated that Niacin (specifically vitamin B3 and also sometimes referred to as nicotinic acid) can raise HDL from 15 to 35 percent. See *www.mayoclinic.com/health/niacin/CL00036*. Niacin decreases your triglyceride and LDL levels, and that's desirable because high levels increase your risk for heart disease. Think of your HDL, or good cholesterol, as a cleanup guy or sanitary worker, because its job is to pick up the excess bad cholesterol from your bloodstream and carry it back to your liver where it gets dumped. Doctors recommend niacin as a treatment for niacin deficiency, high cholesterol, and also high blood fats, or lipids. If your LDL level is high, check with your doctor about taking a niacin supplement (capsule or tablet) to see if you can get your HDL level above 60 milligrams per decilitre—the ideal for both men and women.

110. Take Vitamin C to Protect Against Possible Risk of Certain Cancers

There is growing evidence that vitamin C may have a protective effect in cancers of the esophagus, mouth, pharynx, stomach, pancreas, cervix, rectum, breast, and lung. The most promising evidence, however, is with stomach cancer. High doses of vitamin C in animals inhibit H. pylori, the bacterium that is responsible for most ulcers and possibly an increased risk of stomach cancer. Vitamin C may also protect against cancer by neutralizing free radicals or blocking the formation of nitrosamines. These carcinogenic compounds form when nitrates (found naturally in foods and as food additives) or nitrites (found naturally in saliva) combine with substances called amines in the digestive juices of the stomach.

chapter six
Make Healthy Lifestyle Choices

111. Wander Around a Labyrinth

The ancient labyrinth symbolizes the wandering each of us does with each step we take through our lives. Sometimes the journey features paths that are twisted and confusing. At other times, the road is straight and easy to follow. Walking a labyrinth can be calming to a confused, agitated, or just stressed-out mind. In medieval times, churches with labyrinths were popular among the faithful who used the maze, no doubt, as paths of departure inward to their spiritual centers. Today labyrinthine pattern can be found everywhere, from logos of rock bands on T-shirts to painted patterns on private decks or constructed in pebbles and stones in a backyard garden. You might even see them in gang spray paint graffiti or in tattoos and body art. You can make your own from an old sheet. Study the pictures of historical labyrinths, such as France's Notre Dame Cathedral that you can see on Google images. Walk your labyrinth and ponder your own life's journey and all the great lifestyle and healthy choices you can make to ensure you have the future you desire.

112. Use Music in Your Daily Activities

The notion that music can modulate mood and affect your health in beneficial ways is the basis of an emerging field of study known as music therapy. If music isn't part of your lifestyle, to look and feel younger, why not start listening to music while shopping or exercising or doing other tasks? It can heighten the experience, make the time pass more pleasantly, or reduce the level of stress you might otherwise experience when dealing with a particularly stressful event such as prepping for an audit by the IRS, meeting with your mortgage lender, or anticipating the delivery of bad news. Use your MP3 player or other portable device with some earphones to shut out the stressors in your environment and enjoy music throughout your day.

113. Be a Cooperative and Considerate Driver

How do you deal with feelings of road rage when cars in traffic cut you off, prevent you from moving forward at a green light, or tailgate you? Do you ever mouth obscenities or make obscene gestures to other drivers whose driving style you don't like? To get a handle on your own road rage, think about the possibility that you could stop trying to beat the clock every time you pull out of the driveway. Also, you could focus on things that make the journey pleasurable. For example, listen to a CD of calm, peaceful, uplifting or classical music the next time you're in the car. Give yourself plenty of time to get to your destination. Be a considerate and cooperative driver. Remember that aggressive driving and behaviors trigger those same feelings and behaviors in other drivers.

114. Support Legislation to Label Genetically Altered Foods

Perhaps you embrace an activism lifestyle or perhaps you don't, but a cause that everyone can rally around is the labeling of genetically altered foods. Genetically altered foods started becoming the focus of news stories in the 1990s. While supporters of biotech foods argue that they are safe, others say the full story is not yet known and that without labels on such foods, consumers are not being given a choice about what they put into their bodies. Statistics suggest that as much as 70 percent of U.S. and Canadian processed foods contain genetically modified ingredients (since many contain genetically engineered soy and corn, common ingredients in many packaged food products). Although the countries in the European Union as well as China, New Zealand, Japan, and Australia require mandatory labeling of foods containing genetically altered ingredients, the United States currently does not. Whether or not you believe in the safety of eating genetically altered food, consider supporting legislation for labeling such items because it enables consumers on both sides of the issue to make informed choices about the food they eat.

115. Think of Food as a Lifestyle Choice

Your heart and blood vessels are responsible for transporting oxygen- and glucose-rich blood to all parts of your body. Impaired or damaged heart and blood vessels can't get enough oxygen or glucose to the brain and that will impact anybody's lifestyle. Coronary heart disease is easier to prevent than it is to treat, especially if you have a family history of heart problems, because you can take pre-emptive measures. The keys to holding back coronary heart disease include regular, heart-strengthening exercise (at least four times a week) and a healthful diet low in fat and cholesterol and high in antioxidant-rich fruits and vegetables. Basically, a low-fat diet has less animal protein, very little fried food, and increased amounts of whole grains and vegetables. Be good to your heart, and it will be good to your brain—allowing you to enjoy the activities you love, possibly for the rest of your life.

116. Get Screened for Chlamydia

According to the Centers for Disease Control (CDC), women can get chlamydia, the most frequently sexually transmitted disease (STD) in the United States, and not have symptoms. Chlamydia infection can be transmitted from pregnant mothers to their babies during childbirth (potentially causing neonatal eye and lung problems). Chlamydia infection can also lead to pelvic inflammatory disease. Doctors have long known that pelvic inflammatory disease has been associated with ectopic pregnancy and sterility. Because of the increase in incidents of chlamydia in the last few years and the burden of disease and risks associated with infection, the CDC advocates annual screening of all sexually active women, ages twenty-five and younger for chlamydia. Visit your doctor or local clinic and get screened if you haven't already.

117. Limit High-Fat Foods to Keep Your Brain Young and Healthy

A Canadian study to examine the dietary risk for developing brain changes was published in 2008 on ScienceDirect.com. The study linked a high-fat diet to brain changes akin to those seen in Alzheimer's. The study used mice, ages four to thirteen months, who were fed diets that were formulated to be low in polyunsaturated fats or high in fat. Compared with the control group, the mice fed the high-fat diet showed brain changes as well as weight gain. That scientific study and others like it suggest that food choices clearly affect your brain health and physical well-being. If you have good health, cut out the high-fat foods to ensure that you can continue enjoying optimum brain and body health and the lifestyle you love.

118. Wear a Helmet

It's been estimated that 75 percent of all bicycling deaths result from brain injury. It's the law in many states to wear a helmet when riding a motorcycle. Skateboarding, bicycling, hockey, football, and rock climbing are all sports that encourage participants to wear helmets. If you even suspect that your brain might be susceptible to injury, forgo cool and strap on a helmet. When you fall and hit your head and go unconscious, even though you can't see through your skull, you are likely bruised and bleeding. We now know that if you are unconscious for over an hour from a head injury, you have twice the risk of developing Alzheimer's. After the bleeding stops and the swelling goes down from head trauma, you can still have scar tissue that may be involved in the future development of Alzheimer's.

119. Protect Yourself During Mosquito Season

Mosquitoes are pesky little critters that can infect you with some nasty illnesses, including West Nile virus, malaria, dengue fever, and a host of other undesirable maladies. Experts say that one in ten people are highly attractive to mosquitoes, but they don't understand exactly why. Male mosquitoes, as it turns out, are not the biters—it's the females, and they aren't just hungry and looking for a meal. They need human blood to make their eggs fertile. And the females are attracted to certain compounds found upon your skin, especially if you have high concentrations of cholesterol or steroids on your skin surface, are overweight or pregnant (heavy people and pregnant women give off higher amounts of carbon dioxide), or are moving a lot (like playing tag football or shooting hoops) and generating heat. If you don't want to be a mosquito attractor and, thus, potentially a host to the diseases their bites can trigger, protect yourself with repellant and long-sleeved shirts and trousers. Buy a mosquito net tent for camping or sleeping in rooms in national parks housing, and during visits to places known to have mosquitoes, whether it's a Greek island or a Third World country where windows have no screens.

120. Pay Attention to the Symptoms of Lyme Disease

If you are a nature lover with an active lifestyle, love hiking woodland trails, but don't know what a black-legged tick looks like, you might want to check out the University of Maryland Medical Center's web posting on Lyme disease at *www.umm.edu/patiented/articles/how_ serious_lyme_disease_000016_4.htm.* When a black-legged tick bites you, it transmits a bacterium known as Borrelia burgdorferi, the cause of Lyme disease. The illness reveals itself by headache, fever, fatigue, and a characteristic circular bull's eye skin rash. If caught early, it can be successfully treated with a regimen of antibiotics, but early detection is a key factor. The longer symptoms go untreated, the more likely you will have persistent symptoms and risk having Lyme disease spread to other areas of the body, producing problems such as persistent fatigue, severe arthritis, and decline in cognitive function and mood. If you live in an area where ticks are endemic, apply repellant, wear clothing that covers arms and legs, and check for ticks on your body after outings. If you find a tick, remove it promptly but gently with tweezers.

121. Use Hand Sanitizer During Cold and Flu Season

When the flu comes into your neighborhood, whether it is the Avian flu, the Swine flu, or some other strain or combination of strains, you need to get aggressive to avoid contracting it. Wash your hands often with soap and water and also use hand sanitizer. Take that hand sanitizer with you to restaurants and use it to discretely wipe the table surface before your waitress puts down the dinnerware. The common cold belongs to a family of roughly 200 different viruses and remains viable on a hard surface for hours. Wipe it off. And while you are at it, break the habit of frequently touching your nose, mouth, and eyes where it can be easily introduced into your body.

122. Rethink the Impact of Your Lifestyle on Your Health

Do you donate blood to the Red Cross or other blood banks? Whenever you give blood at a blood bank such as one associated with a university hospital, you will have to go through an intense screening process and will be asked many personal questions about your lifestyle: Have you recently been tattooed? Do you have other body piercings? Do you have unprotected sex? Have you had protected sex with someone who is bisexual? Have you recently traveled to the United Kingdom or Mexico? The answers will reflect the choices you have made in living your life, and those choices will impact the safety of the nation's blood banks. If your blood is unsafe for the critically ill, you may be making choices that could adversely impact your own health. Do an honest evaluation of your behaviors and ask yourself if any of them are risky enough to affect your health. Make adjustments as necessary.

123. Take Care of Your Teeth and Gums

The incidence of dental caries declines as you age, but gum disease including inflammation (gingivitis) or periodontitis, the more severe form of the disease, becomes more commonplace, especially among middle-aged adults. Regular dental checkups continue to be just as important as they were when you were younger. Healthy teeth and gums are important barriers against bacteria that can get into your bloodstream and cause serious illness. Practice good oral hygiene such as regular brushing and flossing to keep dental plaque and bacteria under control. When gums are inflamed and bleeding, you may already be suffering from periodontitis, a condition in which bone loss occurs (below the gum) and the gums begin to recede. It weakens your mouth's ability to defend against disease. Also, more than half of all periodontal disease cases are attributed to smokers, so quit. If you need help quitting, there are ample resources such as patches and even pills.

124. Tune Up Your Chakras

Chakras (the word *chakra* means "wheel" in Sanskrit) are energy vortices or whorls that, according to ancient Indian medicine and yoga philosophy, are aligned along the length of the spine from the tailbone to the top of the head in the subtle etheric body, invisible to the naked eye. There are seven main chakras, and together, they are barometers of health and emotional/mental well-being. When the chakras are all spinning correctly (they each have their own spinning frequency) perfect health ensues; however, too little or too much energy in the body and the imbalance causes ill health. To feel your best, consider having a chakra tune up by a specialist working in alternative medical modalities such as reiki, acupuncture, tai chi, chi kung, or shiatsu massage. You may also be able to shift the energy and tune your chakras through yoga exercises with meditations on light and sound.

125. Give Osteopathic Holistic Medicine a Try

It can be frustrating for a patient to have her doctor treat a health problem and somewhere in the process of interpreting the diagnostic tests, labs, symptoms, and the like, the doctor loses sight of the fact that he's treating a person, not just an illness. If that describes your experience, you might want to consider seeing a doctor trained in osteopathic medicine, a holistic discipline that does not focus purely on the disease but rather the person as well. Osteopathic physicians are licensed and can prescribe medications and give injections as well as perform surgeries. The Princeton Review noted that doctors of osteopathy comprise roughly 6 percent of the workforce of doctors currently practicing in the United States. Their training is based on the philosophy that the human body knows how to cure itself. Their training spans the workings of the musculoskeletal system, holistic medicine principles and practices, and environmental influences and impact, as well as proper nutrition. An osteopathic doctor is not a chiropractor, but rather more like a medical doctor. To find one near you, go to the American Osteopathic Association and type in your information, *www.osteopathic .org/directory.cfm.*

126. Consume a Diet Rich in Flavonols

In a study done by Salk Institute researcher Henriette van Praag and colleagues, a compound found in cocoa—epicatechin—combined with exercise, was found to promote functional changes in a part of the brain involved in the formation of learning and memory. Epicatechin is one of a group of chemicals called flavonols, which have previously been shown to improve cardiovascular function and increase blood flow to the brain. Dr. van Praag's findings, published in the May 30, 2007, issue of *The Journal of Neuroscience,* suggest a diet rich in flavonols could help reduce the effects of neurodegenerative illnesses such as Alzheimer's disease and cognitive disorders related to aging.

127. Savor Dark Chocolate, but Don't Overlook the Prunes

According to study results published in the American Chemical Society's *Journal of Agriculture and Food Chemistry,* cocoa powder has nearly twice the antioxidants of red wine and up to three times what is found in green tea. Although scientists knew that cocoa contains significant antioxidants, they didn't know how rich in antioxidants it is until the Oxygen Radical Absorbance Capacity (ORAC) test examined the antioxidant levels of various foods. The higher the ORAC score, the higher the level of antioxidants present in the food. Based on the U.S. Department of Agriculture/American Chemical Society's findings, dark chocolate tested the highest for antioxidants over other fruits and vegetables. Comparing the levels of antioxidants, dark chocolate came in with a score of 13,120; its closest competitor, milk chocolate, had levels of 6,740; and third was prunes, at 5,770.

128. Breathe to Gather Positive Energy

You can deepen your relaxation using breath by imagining that you are breathing in *prana*, or the positive vital force of life, and exhaling all tension and negative feeling or experience. One way to do this is to choose two colors, one for the prana and one for the negative energy. See a stream of one color (positive) coming into your body as you inhale, and a stream of the other color (negative) flowing out of your body as you exhale. The colors white and black are easy to identify—white is the pure energy of light, and black represents any dark thoughts. But use any colors that you feel represent healing energy and release of negative energy. Don't worry if distracting thoughts arise. Let them float off (you can tell them you will attend to their needs later) like soap bubbles in the air and return to attending to your breathing.

129. Consider the Risks Before Getting Body Piercing and Tattoos

For many young people and those young at heart, body piercing is both a rite of passage and also a deeply personal choice. The Centers for Disease Control (CDC) warn that since artists working within the body art industry depend upon the human body to do their art, the artists are in a unique position to come into contact with their customers' blood. Both individuals who have body piercing and also tattoo artists risk being exposed to certain blood-borne pathogens—hepatitis B virus, hepatitis C virus, or human immunodeficiency virus (HIV). If you want to have your ears, belly button, tongue, eyebrow, or some other body part pierced, practice the following safety tips: Keep the area clean by washing the pierced site often throughout the day with antibacterial soap, and apply a thin coat of antibiotic ointment (too thickly spread and it might encourage the growth of trapped bacteria). For tongue or mouth piercings, stop smoking and using alcohol, and apply a bandage if it helps prevent irritation. For bleeding, apply pressure; for swelling or bruising, place a cold pack wrapped in a clean washcloth over the area. See your doctor if you notice signs of infection or an allergic reaction.

130. Resume Your Workout Routine after Vacation

Sometimes you may get sick. You may go on vacation. You may miss your exercise or weight training workouts for any number of reasons. You're likely to lose some strength during these times. That's normal. Just get right back into your workout schedule. It's the consistency over your lifetime that will pay the most dividends. And, it's easier the second, third, and fourth time around, because your muscles have a "memory." Just don't let them forget for too long. Avoid overtraining and "over-recovery."

131. Use Henna on Hair but Not on Hands

The Food and Drug Administration currently has issued an important alert for henna used in the body-decorating process known as mehndi. Gaining popularity, especially among young women who like the look of a pattern painted on their hands, henna has long been approved by the FDA for coloring the hair. However, henna for skin application necessarily uses a color additive that makes the product unapproved (thus, illegal in the United States). To achieve the dramatic blue or black color, henna may be combined with p-phenylenediamine (approved for use in hair dye) but when used on skin can cause allergic reactions in some people. Visit the FDA's site for more information at *www.fda.gov/Cosmetics.*

132. Find Balance in Your Life

Seek balance between work and play in your life. If you never seem to be able to finish your work, maybe you need to delegate more, get more efficient at what you do, or reorganize and reprioritize your work. To regain balance, take time away from work and worry to just play. Join a friend for a day trip or take the family out to a park or somewhere nice outdoors for a picnic. The fresh air and sunshine will help clear your mind and re-energize your body. The stack of work on your desk will still be there when you get back.

133. Invite a Friend to Help You Get Healthier

You've decided to live a healthier lifestyle, so spread the concept. Get your girlfriends involved. Go shopping together for the ingredients to make a healthy, homemade meal. Enlist one or more friends to help you discover interesting ways to prepare heart-healthy entrees using whole grains, nuts, eggs, legumes, fish, and chicken. Purchase beef, pork, and veal that are certified organic, range fed, and free of additives, and talk with your friends about the reasons why it's the best choice. Use extra virgin olive oil if possible for recipes calling for oil. Remind each other to eschew packaged products over fresh. Split the cost of a cookbook for healthy meals and with your friends, cook something a little spicy, saucy, or just sensational, certain to delight your senses.

chapter seven
Age-Proof Your Brain

134. Exercise Your Brain with Mental Workouts

A 1993 experiment with two groups of mice showed the importance of exercising the brain. The first group was placed in a barren cage with no mental stimulation. They ate, slept, or roamed around the cage. The second group was trained in running complex mazes. After a few weeks, an electron microscope was used to compare the nerve cells of the trained mice to those of the untrained group. The maze mice had developed wider and longer nerve dendrites and more synapses than the mice with no stimulation. In the next phase of the study, the maze group was put in solitary confinement without stimulation. At the end of several more weeks, their brains were examined. They no longer had enhanced dendrites and synapses; they had all shrunken away as if their brains had never been trained. "Use it or lose it" was the conclusion of this study. There are many ways to perform mental workouts to keep your brain fit for life. Try crossword or math puzzles, read a book instead of watching television, if you must watch the tube, choose history documentaries or programs on the Learning Channel that will teach you and work your brain instead of simply watching programs for entertainment.

135. Meet Your Amino Acid Needs

Digestive enzymes break protein down into short amino-acid chains and then finally into individual amino acids. These amino acids can then enter the bloodstream and travel to the cells, where the body rebuilds them into the sequence or into the type of protein that it needs for a specific task. The body continually gets the amino acids it needs from a diet that meets its protein needs and from its own amino-acid pool. In general, animal proteins contain all nine of the essential amino acids and are therefore considered complete proteins. Foods such as legumes, vegetables, grains, nuts, and seeds are considered incomplete proteins because they are missing sufficient quantities of one or more essential amino acids. Eat a balanced diet that includes both animal and plant sources of protein to get the amino acids your body requires from external sources.

136. Memorize Your Grocery List

Enhance your memorization skills at every opportunity and take advantage of the challenges life presents every day. For example, when introduced to someone new, repeat the person's name to yourself three times and use it in conversation. See how well you remember the name the next morning. Another memory trick is to turn a grocery run into a game. After you've made a written list of your needs, memorize it to the best of your ability by taking a mental walk through your kitchen and pantry. Shop without referring to the list and see how well you've done before checking out. If your memory is sharp, you'll probably be able to remember almost everything.

137. Use Chocolate as a Stimulant

One of the best things about chocolate is that "feel good lift" you get after eating a few pieces. It can be attributed to the caffeine present in small quantities or the theobromine, another weak stimulant, present in slightly higher amounts. In any case, the combination of these two, in tandem with the other 298 chemicals present, may just provide the "lift" that makes your day a little better. As a matter of fact, chocolate also contains phenylethylamine, a strong stimulant related to the amphetamine family, known to increase the activity of neurotransmitters in parts of the brain that control your ability to pay attention and stay alert.

138. Write Your Memoir

This can be a very rewarding activity in that you preserve your life experiences for the benefit of other family members and exercise your brain in the process. Recalling previous events requires a strong memory (which may be aided by going through photo albums, letters, old documents, and postcards), and the act of writing improves visual-spatial skills. If you've lived a truly extraordinary life, think of the most dramatic and pivotal moments as scenes in a book or movie. Write your life story without including every mundane detail, but rather as a sequence of dramatic, poignant, heartwrenching, uplifting, momentous, historical, and relevant scenes. Why not consider getting your memoir published?

139. Choose a Hobby That Stimulates Different Parts of Your Brain

According to Daniel G. Amen, MD, in *Making a Good Brain Great*, it's far better to learn something new than to repeat the same activities: "The best mental exercise is acquiring new knowledge and doing things that you haven't done before . . . when the brain does something over and over, even a complicated task, it learns how to do it using less and less energy." Find a hobby that requires coordination between multiple brain regions, such as ballroom dancing, painting, or learning a musical instrument. Knitting, photography, woodworking, gardening, writing poetry, or anything that requires you to study something new will also stimulate your brain. Don't take the easy way out either; pick something that challenges you and then strive to do it well. All of these activities will strengthen and maintain mental acuity on a variety of levels.

140. Learn to Speak Spanish

Being multilingual is extremely beneficial these days, and learning a foreign language can also be quite mentally challenging because it requires the thoughtful assimilation of new information and a strong memory. Struggle with those verbs, pore over grammatical structure, force yourself to speak it at every opportunity, and stick with it even when it seems futile. The minute it feels like your brain is stretching, you're already succeeding. Once you've learned a new language, reward yourself with a vacation to the country where it is spoken so you can practice the new language and learn more about its culture.

141. Support Brain Function with Rainforest Medicinal Plants

Increasingly, scientists and medical researchers seek to discover and understand the medicinal properties of rainforest herbs and flora, perhaps especially those that could be beneficial in treating cancer, immunological problems, and illnesses of the brain. In fact, one popular brain-support nutritional supplement, Amazon Brain Support from Raintree, lists ten Amazon rainforest botanicals in its formulation, including samambaia, calaguala, tamamuri, catuaba, muira puama, cat's claw, suma, guarana, nettle, and sarsaparilla. Rainforest plants are complex chemical storehouses that contain many undiscovered biodynamic compounds with unrealized potential for use in modern medicine. Following are some of the most important healing medicinal plants, as listed in *Herbal Secrets of the Rainforest* by Leslie Taylor. You can also learn more by reading *Kava: Medicine Hunting in Paradise* by Chris Kilham, who conducts research on medicinal plants around the world.

Cat's Claw—Aids intestinal immune system and chronic arthritis.
Damiana—Used for hormone regulation in men and women.
Guarana—Promotes health and energy.
Muira Puama—Relieves stress; regulates hormones; promotes healthy central nervous system; general health tonic.
Suma—Regulates female hormones; strengthens immune system; aids in regulation of cholesterol. Also used as general health tonic. Also known as Brazilian ginseng.

142. Play the Violin, the Orchestra's Most Difficult Instrument

According to Daniel G. Amen, author of *Making a Good Brain Great,* the College Entrance Examination Board in 1996 reported that students with experience in musical performance scored 51 points higher on the verbal part of the SAT and 39 points higher on the math section than the national average. In another study, music majors were the most likely group of college grads to be admitted to medical school (66 percent, the highest percentage of any group). If you want more brain power, go to a music store or your nearest music lesson studio and try out some different instruments. Some music stores rent instruments such as violins, cellos, flutes, trumpets, and clarinets on a monthly basis. That way you aren't stuck with an instrument if you find it isn't to your liking. Take lessons and practice a lot—it'll be good for your brain.

143. Connect the Alfalfa/Brain Nutrient Dots

Modern scientists have discovered that alfalfa is rich in minerals and other nutrients, including calcium, magnesium, potassium, and beta-carotene, and may reduce "bad" cholesterol. Alfalfa leaf is on the FDA's list of herbs generally regarded as safe, but it should be used in medicinal amounts only with your doctor's approval. Besides containing nutrients and minerals that benefit the body and brain, alfalfa can be an agent in the treatment of heart disease, stroke, and cancer—the top three causes of death in the United States. Eat the leaves or sprouts in salads or put through a juicer with other raw vegetables for a healthy drink. If you experience any side effects—such as upset stomach or diarrhea—stop use. **Caution:** Alfalfa seeds are to be avoided entirely, especially by anyone with an autoimmune problem.

144. Learn to Play Chess

According to Dr. Frank Lawlis in *The IQ Answer*, an idle brain loses brainpower. Engage your brain. Play bridge, chess, poker, bingo, and charades. Mensa (an organization of brainiacs, those who rank in the top 2 percent when it comes to IQ), favor playing brain stimulation games such as Brainstrain, Cityscape, Cube Checkers, Doubles Wild, and Finish Lines. Many more can be found in the American Mensa Library.

145. Sign Up for a Memorization Class

Research has proved the success of training and practice when it comes to maintaining and strengthening our mental abilities. In one study, scientists evaluated the number of words people could recall after listening to a lengthy list of random words. Before they received memory training, the older members of the study group were able to recall fewer words than the younger members. But after just a handful of memory-training sessions, which included tips such as placing words in meaningful groups (for example, using the mnemonic "Every Good Boy Does Fine" to recall the musical notes on the staff lines—E G B D F) rather than trying to memorize them out of context, the older participants were able to triple their word recall. Many sites on the Internet offer memorization classes and you may even find some courses at your local community college or through parks and recreation department offerings. But here's another idea: make a deck of flashcards using English or foreign-language words to be memorized. You could also use scriptural verses, poems, songs, or speeches such as

Lincoln's Gettysburg Address. Write or type it, print, and glue to a card. In a quiet room, read the first sentence and memorize it. Close your eyes and repeat it aloud. Do the same for the second sentence. Repeat the first and second sentences aloud . . . and so forth. If you become tired, have a light snack, but stay with it. When you have completed your session, take a nap. Although the memory is still fragile, scientific study has shown that there is a greater likelihood that you'll retain the new memory if you take a nap right after your brain workout.

146. Try Sage and Lemon Balm Extract to Improve Your Memory

Professor Elaine Perry, of the University of Newcastle upon Tyne in northern England, told members of a medical conference on the psychiatry of old age held in February 2004 that the plant extracts of sage and lemon balm produced promising results in studies to improve memory and behavior in Alzheimer's patients. Dr. Perry said: "In controlled trials in normal volunteers, both extracts improved memory, and lemon balm improved mood. Lemon balm reduced agitation and improved quality of life in people with Alzheimer's disease." Use lemon balm and sage in aromatherapy. Or, take the herbs in tablets, teas, tinctures, capsules, essential oils, and extracts.

147. Limit the Television Watching and Engage Your Brain

Some people become numbed—mentally and physically—by watching too much television. Others dull their brains with alcohol and other stupefying substances. Prescription and over-the-counter drug interactions can also impair cognitive function, as can certain medical conditions. But for the majority of older Americans, isolation and a lack of social interaction are the primary culprits. Social support involves a lot of social interaction and includes chatting with friends, engaging in a variety of activities, and living a relatively active life. All of this stimulates the brain on a number of important levels, keeping your cognitive skills well honed. But older people who lack social support often have little to do to occupy their time except watch television. Opportunities to actually think, to exercise the brain, become increasingly limited. And with this lack of stimulation comes a subtle but serious reduction in mental functioning.

148. Take Primrose Capsules for Brain Health

Evening primrose oil is high in linoleic acid and has been shown to help lower blood cholesterol, which is good for your circulatory system, and thus good for your brain. The usual dose is one 250-milligram capsule three times a day. Swedish studies, though preliminary, relate evening primrose oil to an antioxidant that counteracts the formation of free radicals, which are especially active in the aging process.

149. Try Ginkgo Biloba to Improve Memory and Cognition

The leaves of the ginkgo contain the active constituents ginkgo flavone glycosides and terpene lactones, the extract of which can be used to treat poor circulation in the legs as well as memory and cognitive problems. In a study published in the *Journal of the American Medical Association,* researchers confirmed that people who take the ginkgo extract for mild to severe dementia may improve both their ability to remember and to interact socially. Usual daily dosage for the extract is 120 to 240 milligrams in three doses. Plan to take it for at least eight weeks before improvement shows. For capsules, take the same amount daily as recommended above. The standard capsule contains 40 to 60 milligrams. Buy a quality product and read the label. Look for products marked "24/6," an indication the product contains 24 percent flavone glycosides and 6 percent terpenes. Note, however, the caveat for taking ginkgo: Although it is considered a brain-friendly herb, for reasons scientists don't understand, ginkgo may interfere with antidepressant MAO-inhibitor drugs such as phenelzine sulfate (Nardil) or tranylcypromine (Parnate). If you're on heart medication and want to take ginkgo, consult your doctor first.

150. Avoid Brain Atrophy

The hippocampus is the part of your brain essential for learning and remembering new information, but what you eat and how you deal with stress could impact the health of your hippocampus. Research has shown that consuming the typical American-style diet along with sustained stress can damage that part of the brain. Researchers at the University of South Florida's James A. Haley Veterans Administration Medical Center and Arizona State University found that chronically stressed rats consuming an American-style diet of excessive carbohydrates and beef fat experienced atrophy of the hippocampus. Rats fed a high-fat diet and living under chronic stress (living in crowded conditions, in close proximity to cats) developed hippocampal atrophy, expressed in reduced dendrite length. Dendrites are the connections between brain cells where information is stored. The researchers deduced that the combination of a high-fat diet and stress can interfere with the ability of the brain—in rats or people—to learn new information. Previous research had shown that rats on a high-fat diet produce an excessive amount of corticosterone in response to stress. Corticosterone, a steroid hormone produced by the adrenal glands, can also damage the hippocampus, indicating that a high-fat diet and stress are doubly detrimental to the brain. Start age-proofing your brain by reducing the stressors in your environment and choosing foods loaded with brain nutrients such as fish, nuts, and blueberries, for example, instead of marbled cuts of steak, greasy burgers and fries, and high-fat snacks.

151. Eat Whole Grains to Nutritionally Power Your Brain

Foods made from grains should be the base of a nutritious diet if you want to boost your brain power through the foods you eat. The ancient Romans had a saying, *mens sana in corpora sano* (a healthy mind in a healthy body). Grains include corn, wheat, rice, and oats. Whole-grain foods supply vitamin E and B vitamins such as folic acid as well as minerals like magnesium, iron, and zinc. Whole grains (like whole wheat) are rich in fiber and higher in other important nutrients that can make their way to your brain. Eating plenty of whole-grain breads, bran cereals, and other whole-grain foods also can easily provide half of your fiber needs for an entire day. When choosing grains look for the words *whole grain* or *whole wheat* to make sure the product is made from 100 percent whole wheat flour. The aim should be to consume at least six servings of grain products per day. Choose grains that are rich in fiber, low in saturated fat, and low in sodium.

152. Try Gotu Kola Brain Food

Because the ancient herb gotu kola helps rebuild energy reserves, it has become known as "food for the brain." Supposed to increase mental and physical strength, combat stress, and improve reflexes, it is popular in the West as a nerve tonic. Recent studies have shown that it improves circulation by increasing the flow of blood throughout the body and strengthening veins and capillaries. It is typically taken as capsules or an extract; follow the label's directions. Pregnant woman should not use this herb, nor should anyone with an overactive thyroid condition.

153. Understand Macronutrients

The brain is only a fraction of the total weight of the body, about 2 percent, but requires 20 percent of the body's blood supply, 20 percent of the body's total oxygen supply, and 65 percent of its glucose. Along with the rich supply of glucose, the brain needs a host of other nutrients. Nutrients are grouped into six different categories:

carbohydrates, proteins, fats, vitamins, minerals, and water. Carbo-hydrates, proteins, and fats are called macronutrients because we need larger amounts in our diet. Some foods consist of one, two, or all three of these macronutrients. Even though each macronutrient has a particular function in the body, they work in partnership for good health. Our bodies need all three macronutrients to function properly, but not in equal amounts. Some evidence suggests that a diet with macronutrients in the wrong proportions is a risk factor for diseases like coronary heart disease and certain cancers.

154. Make Nutrition a Priority

Nutrition, perhaps more than any other factor, plays an essential role in your overall health, including brain function and longevity. The reason for this is simple: The foods you eat affect virtually every cell, organ, and system in your body. If you eat enough of the right foods, your body thrives, and you will live well and long. According to nutrition experts, a healthful diet provides your cells with every-thing they need to function well, reproduce, and repair damage from a variety of sources. Healthful foods also give your body the right kind of fuel so that you have plenty of energy and a strong immune system. But there's more. The right kinds of foods help your body get rid of waste products and potentially harmful toxins, many of which can increase your risk of serious illness, including cancer, if not purged regularly. And they help reduce your risk of many chronic disorders commonly associated with aging, includ-ing osteoporosis and heart disease.

155. Eat Chicken Vindaloo

Scientists at the University of California in Los Angeles have done laboratory studies on the association of curcumin, a chemical found in curry spices and tumeric—used in cooking chicken vindaloo—and amyloid-beta, the substance that causes plaques in the brains of Alzheimer disease patients. The researchers noted that curcumin may assist the immune system in ridding the brain tissue of amyloid-beta plaques. Turmeric (*Curcuma longa*) also has a beneficial effect on digestion; it stimulates the flow of bile and the breakdown of dietary fats. More scientific research is needed, but with what is already known about curcumin, it appears that you may gain some brain benefit by eating foods made with curry spices, especially turmeric.

156. Drink Skim Milk

Skim milk has lower fat, but perhaps equally important, it has abundant choline. Upping your choline intake may improve memory and stave off senility. Choline is an essential building block of all cells. For over ten years, scientists have been studying the effect of choline supplementation in rat brains, specifically on memory. Their findings showed that the rats that prenatally got adequate amounts of choline did not appear to develop senility as they aged. And, human studies showed that increasing the intake of choline can improve memory and cognitive functioning. Eating egg yolks, if you don't have elevated cholesterol, and drinking skim milk could make nutritional sense currently and pay big dividends later in life.

chapter eight

Get a Good Night's Sleep

157. Instead of Popping a Pill, Eat a High-Carbohydrate Snack

A bedtime snack of toast with jam or fruit and crackers can trigger the release of serotonin, a brain chemical that aids in sleep. Toast and peanut butter does the trick for some people while a light snack of crackers with a glass of warm milk helps others to more easily drift off to sleep. Evaluate your lifestyle and food intake and see if you can find the culprits of dreaded insomnia—for example, a heavy caloric meal at dinner, foods that are too spicy and may bring on heartburn at bedtime, or habitually getting up during the night for snacks and thus rewarding your stomach and establishing a bad habit. Eat a light, balanced dinner and a high-carbohydrate small snack before bed. You may find it easier to fall asleep and stay asleep.

158. Know If You Are Getting Enough Sleep

Doctors suggest that on average most people need six to eight hours of sleep each night. But not everyone gets it. Insomnia is one of the most prevalent problems in the United States, and one of the most common reasons people visit a doctor. It's estimated that one in four American adults and one in two seniors experience occasional or recurrent sleep problems, and those figures will continue to rise as the baby boomer generation reaches old age. Sleep disturbances—more commonly known by the umbrella term "insomnia"—can be caused by a host of reasons, including depression and chronic pain, but a hectic lifestyle is probably the most common.

159. Understand the Pitfalls of Sleep Deprivation

Sleep disturbances are more than a minor inconvenience; severe, chronic insomnia can have a devastating effect on physical and mental well-being, which in turn can have a dramatic influence on aging. Even occasional insomnia can affect your health to some degree, including a weakening of the immune system. Some research suggests that chronic sleep deprivation can shorten the years of your life. So if you want to get rid of those dark circles or bags under your eyes, maintain a healthy body and strong immune system, and maximize your lifespan, do whatever it takes to get as much daily sleep as your body and brain need.

160. Sleep on the Airplane

When traveling, get the sleep you need. Traveling across different time zones coupled with jet lag can adversely affect your ability to fall asleep and to stay asleep. Sleep experts say that nighttime sleep is divided roughly into five stages of either deeper or lighter sleep and those stages keep shifting. The rapid eye movement (REM) that characterizes muscle relaxation and dreaming occurs toward morning. When you suffer from periods of insomnia, sleep's restorative value is lost or diminished. When you are packing for your trip, take along earplugs, a mask, and a travel pillow and blanket. Try sleeping on the plane instead of typing, chatting, or reading.

161. Take Kava Kava Before Going to Bed

If you've had a stressful day, try some kava. The herb, also known as kava kava, is derived from a rootstock native to the Pacific Islands, where its use is primarily ceremonial and spiritual. It is said to bring "oneness of body and mind." Now sold as a relaxant and anxiety-relieving herb, it first appeared in Europe in the 1860s. In the 1920s, German pharmacists sold kava as a mild sedative and tension reliever. Consumed at bedtime as a tea, it promotes restful sleep. Kava is found in products with proprietary names such as Jakava, Kava-Phyton, Kavacur, Kavasol, Sedalint Kava, and Songha Day as well as in multi-ingredient products. Caution: Make certain your doctor knows about any herbal supplements or teas that you may be taking as they can interact with other medications and impact existing medical conditions.

162. Limit Your Intake of Caffeine

One of the world's most popular drugs, caffeine is a stimulant that affects the central nervous system, the digestive tract, and metabolism. Caffeine is found in coffee beans, tea leaves, cocoa beans, and products derived from these sources. It is absorbed quickly in the body and can raise blood pressure, heart rate, and brain seratonin levels (low levels of seratonin cause drowsiness). Withdrawal from caffeine can cause headaches and drowsiness. The pharmacological active dose of caffeine is defined as 200 milligrams, and the recommended not-to-exceed daily intake level is the equivalent of one to three cups of coffee (139 to 417 milligrams). Too much caffeine also prematurely ages your brain because it dehydrates and reduces blood flow, and tricks you into thinking you don't need more sleep.

163. De-Stress Before Bed Each Night

After a long day at work, are you tense and restless before falling asleep? Release stress before you go to sleep and you may find that you are able to fall asleep more quickly, have a better quality of sleep, and wake up more rested and refreshed. There are myriad ways to calm your mind and let go of the tension held in your body, including taking a warm bath, sipping a glass of warm milk, listening to relaxation tapes or peaceful music, doing some deep breathing, or praying to release concerns to a higher power. Rather than living your life stressed out, make it a point to let go of the worry and tension accumulated throughout the day so that you get deep, restorative sleep.

164. Maintain a Healthy Lifestyle for Relaxing Sleep

This means eating right and exercising regularly. But sleep specialists warn that you should not exercise immediately before bedtime. Physical activity tends to stimulate the body rather than relax it. If you can, try to work in your exercise in the morning, at lunch, or after work. Evening workouts are okay, but do them several hours before bedtime, so that you have time to wind down. You might try some stretching, a hot soak in the tub, and a warm glass of milk (contains the essential amino acid L-tryptophan that promotes sleep) as part of your bedtime ritual. When it is time to crawl in bed, you'll be relaxed and ready for a good night's sleep.

165. Establish a Sleep Schedule

Determine the best time for you to go to sleep. Understand that you may need a different amount of sleep than someone else. It varies from person to person. You need to understand how much sleep you need to feel rested and alert the next day. Try to go to bed at exactly that time every evening. A soothing bedtime ritual can also help.

166. Use Your Bed Only for Sleep

Watching TV, reading, and eating are best done in the living room—not the bedroom. The goal is to quickly prepare your body for sleep when you finally go to bed. If you find that you haven't fallen asleep within twenty minutes, get up and do something else, such as reading. The movement of your eyes back and forth across the page when reading is similar to the way your eyes move during the REM (rapid eye movement) phase of sleep (as opposed to the non-REM phase). During the REM phase a sound sleeper may rouse out of sleep only to fall back into a deeper sleep whereas the light sleeper may awaken and not be able to fall back to sleep. According to sleep researchers, as you age, your sleep patterns change. Elderly people can have problems getting and staying asleep because of health issues, whereas women can experience sleep disruptions due to menstrual cycles, pregnancy, or menopause.

167. Make Sure Your Bed Is Comfortable

A mattress may make all the difference in how you sleep. A bed that is too hard or too soft can have a serious effect on your ability to fall asleep and stay asleep. When shopping for a new mattress, check out as many different kinds as you can before making your decision. Never buy the first mattress you see, and never buy a mattress without lying on it for several minutes to determine how it feels.

168. Sleep in a Dark, Quiet Room with the Right Temperature

Many people sleep poorly because their bedroom is too noisy, too bright, too hot, or too cold. Some people can sleep under almost any conditions, but most of us need darkness and comfort for a truly restful night's sleep. Soundproof your bedroom if you're bothered by outside noise and use blackout curtains to keep out intrusive light. And don't forget the small things; the light from a seemingly harmless clock face can inhibit sleep in light-sensitive individuals.

169. Don't Linger in Bed after the Alarm Goes Off

Hitting the snooze button every morning can wreak havoc with your internal clock and make you feel tired and listless all day long. Establishing a set time to get up each morning keeps your body clock in sync and ensures restful sleep. Train yourself to get up within a few minutes after the alarm sounds and step into your day. If you need to sit on the side of the bed and wake up your feet and legs, dangle them off the side and turn them in large circles and then smaller ones. By the time they hit the floor, you should be ready to walk into your day.

170. Avoid Alcohol, Tobacco, and Middle-of-the-Night Snacks

Alcohol may make you drowsy, but it interferes with brain activity and can impair sleep. Nicotine is a powerful stimulant; it's the last thing you need if you suffer from insomnia. Skip those really late-night snacks, too. A stomach full of food can interfere with sleep by forcing the body to work when it should be resting. In addition, greasy foods can cause indigestion.

171. Establish Regularity in Your Sleep Patterns

Your body, including your brain, actually mends and maintains itself when you sleep. If you strength train or do any sort of resistance exercise, then your muscles repair themselves and grow stronger when you're asleep. If you don't sleep, your muscles will stay fatigued and not get stronger. Getting enough sleep helps keep you safe; being sleep-deprived increases the likelihood of accidents and mistakes. It's helpful to first recognize that you want to sleep well, i.e., seven to nine hours of uninterrupted sleep each night. Go to sleep and wake up at the same times. Your body loves regularity. If you are someone who sleeps very late on the weekends and then has trouble waking up for work on Monday, or if you sometimes stay up late and then crash the next evening, you aren't helping yourself. Instead, seek regularity in your sleeping patterns.

172. Change Your Breathing Pattern

When you fall asleep, your breathing continues. But if you have respiratory problems or breathing issues such as sleep apnea or snoring, you might be apprehensive about falling asleep. Breath, like food, nourishes your cells and cleanses your blood. However, most people don't take the deep, full breaths they should every day, depriving themselves of the vital nutrient that deep breathing provides. The good news is that changing breathing patterns is easy. Anyone can do it. You first must become aware of your breathing pattern in order to change it. As you lie in bed and prepare to fall asleep, concentrate on your breath. Breathe deeply. Count your breaths as you inhale four and exhale six or eight. Focus on your breath and you may find drifting off to sleep is easier.

173. Curb Worrywart Tendencies

It is well known that a persistent fear or worry will deplete an individual's vitality; it will cause him to feel out of sorts, below par, or not himself. Worrying can interfere with sleep, and chronic worrying can cause the body to lose its natural resistance to disease and become more vulnerable to opportunistic infections and illnesses. Excessive, habitual worrying also keeps your brain unnaturally occupied with fear and dread. That, in turn, taxes your entire body—particularly your brain. You can train your brain to think positively and, with enough redirection of the internal dialogue, you can improve your health, your outlook on life, your energy, and your brain. That self-correction will enable you to get the sleep and rest you need.

174. Focus on Pleasant Experiences in Your Life

A good technique for moving your thoughts away from worry and fear in order to focus on something positive is to think about what you love about your life. Doing so will enable your emotional brain to fire up. Write out five things you're grateful for today. Focus on what is making you feel lucky and good about your life. This trains your brain to focus on the love and pleasant experiences in your life. Do it long enough and you'll effectively create a positive groove in your brain that will create ripple effects in your life. To get to sleep more easily, try lying in bed at night and consciously breathe away the negative energy you've accumulated during the day and then focus on the pleasant experiences in your life.

175. Try St. John's Wort

This herb might lift your spirits if you're feeling down, and may also help you sleep. According to Michael T. Murray, ND, author of *Natural Alternatives to Prozac,* about twenty-five supervised, double-blind studies involving a total of 1,592 patients who received positive effects from St. John's wort reported that it improved psychological problems like depression, anxiety, and sleep disorders without side effects. In his book *Herbs for Your Health,* herbalist Stephen Foster warns that St. John's wort should primarily be used as a safer, non-addictive antidepressant aid until the true causes of the depression are uncovered and treated properly. **Caution:** No one ever should treat depression lightly, and neither St. John's wort nor other herbal treatments should be used to replace prescription drugs being taken by people who have been diagnosed with clinical depression. Do not combine it with antidepressants and always consult your physician first.

176. Learn Self-Hypnosis to Banish Chronic Stress

If you suffer from chronic stress, chances are good that you aren't sleeping well and your lack of deep, nourishing sleep is taking a toll on your health. An October 2000 *Brain Research Bulletin* study confirmed what has been known since the mid-1980s: Cortisol levels are high in Alzheimer's patients. This study also showed that high levels of cortisol correlated with a more rapid deterioration of brain function as evaluated by the Mini-Mental State Examination (a thirty-point questionnaire used to screen for dementia) over a forty-month period in a group of elderly women. It is well known that chronic stress elevates cortisol levels, which is one of the main causes of brain cell death. Popular stress reduction techniques include self-hypnosis, regular prayer, and meditation.

177. Sleep in a Cool Room with Covers

Winter is a time to get out those extra covers or down comforters for warmth in much of America, whereas summer bedding might be no more than a sheet. If you are too hot or too cold when you are sleeping, regardless of the season, the discomfort you feel certainly can cause you to awaken. Sometimes it's not going to sleep but going back to sleep that is at the heart of a person's sleep problems. Many people sleep better in a room with the temperature set a little on the cool side. Put on or take off the covers and set your furnace and air conditioner accordingly. Also, make sure your pillows are not what are causing you to wake up. People with respiratory ailments often need more than one pillow, but otherwise one or two should suffice. If your pillow is too fluffy, hard, soft, flat, or just plain old, try a different pillow until you get the right support and a good night's sleep.

178. Put Unresolved Conflict to Bed First

If you have unresolved issues, it's a good bet that you aren't going to easily fall asleep, but even if you do, you may be waking up throughout the night worrying about them. A phobia is an unreasonable, compulsive, persistent fear. Having to face something you fear can produce a phobia anxiety attack with associated symptoms such as heart palpitations, breathlessness, weakness, an uncontrollable feeling of terror, and even hysterical screaming. Anxiety and phobias are closely related, and both can produce stress. Without resolution, the stress becomes chronic. Get professional help to confront severe unresolved issues causing phobia or anxiety attacks, otherwise, deal with whatever bugs you so that you can get the rest your body requires.

chapter nine

Lighten Up

179. Do Belly Breathing

"Belly" breathing is abdominal or diaphragmatic breathing. When air is taken in, the diaphragm contracts and the abdomen expands; when air is exhaled, the reverse occurs. You can test yourself for abdominal breathing by laying your hand on your belly as you breathe. If it expands as you inhale, you are breathing with the diaphragm. If it flattens, you are breathing with the chest. To practice abdominal breathing, imagine that your inward breath is filling a balloon in your belly. When the balloon is full, exhale until you feel it is completely empty. Just a few of these deep abdominal breaths will bring relief from tension—and pain is half tension. By slowing the breath and thought, you experience tranquility and happiness.

180. Change Your Environment

Consider the role your work day environment may have on your stress level. Think about what you might change in your office, cubicle, or other work site that could help you relax and feel more serene. Could you increase or decrease the lighting, turn up or turn down the thermostat, open a door or window, put up a poster with a pleasing nature scene, or close a door to mute unwanted noise? Make the necessary adjustments that allow you to feel good when you are at work, whether it's a corporate setting or a home office. Anything you can do to reduce your stress level will benefit your body and mind.

181. Take a Mental Health Day

Sometimes you just need to change things up a little. Change the scenery. Change the pace. Change your routine. Not taking a mental health day when you are laboring under the deadline of a stressful job and a heavy work load can be detrimental not only to your body but to your mental and emotional well-being. Your productivity drops when you are mentally and physically exhausted. Give yourself the gift of time. What would you do if you didn't have to be anywhere or do anything? Break your routine and take a day or two or a week, if you need it. Get away from work stress, deadlines, and other job-related challenges and difficulties.

182. Take Your Vacation and Long Weekend Breaks

If you want to be healthier, happier, less moody, and more productive, take a vacation. Resist the urge to take a "working" vacation where the family may cavort on the beach and visit museums while you remain in the hotel working on one or more projects that you brought along. That's missing the purpose of taking time to rest, relax, recuperate, recharge, and renew your body and mind. Some psychologists recommend taking regular time off to reduce burnout from job and family stresses. If you can't afford a long vacation, consider scheduling in some long weekends (three to four days) several times a year to strengthen family bonds and establish a better balance between work and play.

183. De-Stress at Your Desk with Simple Stretches

Consider how many times during the workday that you feel irritable, tense, or highly stressed over something a coworker says or a job that your boss just passed off to you. In both instances, you may feel as if you've just been sucker punched. If you just let all the assaults of the day accumulate, by the end of the day most likely your brain feels fried and your body old and stiff. To release tension and feel a little lighter, remind yourself that unless you give someone else the power to dictate how you feel—and why would you do that—no one can take away your mental and physical well-being. Take a moment to reconnect with whatever makes you feel grounded. Inhale deeply and stretch your arms over your head. Imagine stressful energy racing along your unseen meridians, out of your fingers into the air, and far away from you. Bend side to side, breathing slowly and easily. Lift your legs and lower them several times, imagining stress flowing out of you. Find ways to de-stress, lighten up, and remain calm, yet creative, while doing your job.

184. Shift Your Perspective

Time offers the gift of perspective, but sometimes you just have to adjust the way you think about a situation or circumstance in present time. Shifting your perspective means you can put a small crisis in a larger frame and view it differently. Being able to see that it isn't such a big deal can enable you to view potential ways the crisis might resolve itself. You can stop being so harsh with yourself and instead practice self-appreciation. Treat yourself with love, dignity, and respect, the way you would your lover or best friend.

185. Move On

You've dealt with a crisis—an argument, divorce, death, or some other type of pivotal event. Now let it go. When it's over, move on. Release the tension through breath work, therapy, grief counseling, or some other modality. Seek out that special place inside yourself where you can feel peace and joy at the miracle of being alive and out of harm's way. Do deep breathing to get centered. Engage in mindfulness. You are greater than the sum parts of your body. Let your mind embrace expansiveness. Crisis and its aftermath can make you feel old. Learn to reconnect to the youthful self inside you.

186. Establish and Enforce Personal Boundaries

If you are one of those people who has trouble establishing and enforcing personal boundaries, consider the power of the word "no." It has a purpose and place in every life. If you haven't established personal boundaries, people can take advantage of your kindness and you may unwittingly allow them to either use you or waste your time. When that happens, you get angry at them and perhaps also at yourself, and that's counterproductive. Ensure that you have firm personal boundaries in place and reinforce them with a "no" as necessary. For example, if someone is always interrupting you at work to chat about nonwork topics, establish a boundary. Insist that the door to your office is to be considered closed when you are working and that visitors need to knock first. Remind anyone who violates your rule. If they enter and start chatting, tell them "no, not now." In the long run, having personal boundaries in place can help you lighten up by ensuring that your work is not interrupted, you don't feel angry at others and yourself, and that you are empowered to set and hold firmly in place your own rules.

187. Forgive Old Hurts

If you are still holding on to anger or hurt instead of forgiving the person who violated you, you are limiting your capacity to feel good. Many great religious and spiritual traditions address the issue of forgiveness, reminding us that at our sacred center or core, we are inherently happy. When we hang on to resentment, pain, or anger from the past and recall it in the future, we hurt ourselves. Some yoga teachers have even suggested a connection between a tendency to hold on to resentment and bitterness and the development of heart problems. Don't close down your heart and your feelings. Overcome those negative emotions. Whenever you slip into a place of pain and sadness, say a blessing for yourself. Then say a blessing for the person who hurt you. Tell her that you will no longer take her or the memory of that incident any further into your life. Forgive, bless, and release. That's the way to keep your heart open and your mind and body young.

188. Use Self-Deprecating Humor to Diffuse Hostility

Tense or hostile situations can erupt anywhere and at any time, for example, on the road, in a parking lot, at your workplace, or in line at the movie theater. Someone feels slighted, hurt, angry, defensive, or sick and takes it out on you. It is not always easy to diffuse the tension in such hostile moments. If the person with the problem is someone you know and is verbally accosting you, try using an apology and a little self-deprecating humor to diffuse the tension. Poking fun at yourself may help ease away the other person's aggression.

189. Follow Three Steps to Regain Control over Your Life

When you feel disempowered over some aspect of your life, you become miserable and wonder how things got so crazy. Regaining control over a life that's gotten way too haywired will require that you take at least three steps: become more self-oriented so that your needs are put first; establish and enforce your personal boundaries and stop saying "yes" to everyone for everything; and give yourself the gift of time and perspective to evaluate each problem or area to see what can be done to regain control (and thus, your sanity).

190. Explore the Space Between the Breaths

When you feel as if life has become a kind of prison and you're stuck, not able to move in any direction, take heart. That is precisely the time when you can finally remain quiet, sink into awareness of your inward and outward breathing cycles, and allow your mind to dive deeply into the space between the breaths. That is a very potent place of stillness and calm. There you experience yourself in a whole new way, beyond body and even the consciousness of your mind. As the breath slows, thinking slows as well. You experience a sense of limitless boundaries. From that place of peace, if you allow your mind to formulate a clear question, you will often receive an inspired, intuitive answer.

191. Live Life More Spontaneously

Grant yourself permission to have more freedom and liberty, to live your life more spontaneously from your heart. See happiness not as a destination where you will one day arrive, but rather as a process in the journey of life. Remind yourself to lighten up, notice the images of beauty that are all around you, and feel the healing power of joy. When you choose to see life with that mindset, you begin to open yourself to more happiness and less of all the other emotions that pull you down, restrict your thinking, and curtail any childlike sense of adventure and wonder.

192. Put a Troubling Moment into Perspective

Be thankful that you will never have to live that upsetting moment ever again. It was only a moment in a lifetime of moments . . . not even a day in your life. Whenever something triggers the memory of it, focus on how good you feel now that time and perspective have enabled your to release all feeling associated with it. Make it a goal to see the experience as a gain in terms of what you have learned. Even if you feel steamrolled by some conflict or confrontation with another person, keep the whole situation in perspective. Don't expend any more energy on it. Learn what you can and move on. Constantly rehashing it doesn't help clear those negative feelings. Forgive and move on.

193. Think of Friends as Your Dearest Treasures

If your greatest treasures are members of your family, also think of your friends as your dearest treasures and do whatever you can to safeguard your friendships. Even if you have almost come to blows over some issue (for example, a business dealing with a friend or a difference of opinion about something), take a deep breath and ask yourself if the business deal or the difference of opinion is worth throwing away all the years of that friendship. Chances are likely that the friendship is worth more than the business deal. Hang on to your friends; they are not so easily replaced.

194. Get Your Hair Done to Feel Lighter and Happier

The effects of aging can be seen not only in your face, but also in your hair. Oil glands in the scalp begin to dry out as you grow older, causing your hair to become brittle and more easily broken. White or graying hair occurs when the hair cells gradually stop producing pigment. Researchers have found that nearly half of men and women of European descent will have at least some noticeable graying by age fifty. Others can expect to see graying about a decade later, if not before. Nearly half of all men can expect some balding by their fiftieth birthday. Some will choose to shave their heads—very popular and sexy now. Both men and women also can color their hair with natural products, and a new hairstyle or cut can give you a whole new look as well.

195. Use Mediation to Deal with Hostility

If you ever are in a situation, such as a legal conflict, where there seems to be no apparent resolution to the troubling impasse you have reached, and you desperately seek closure, consider the mediation option. Mediation by an impartial third party can save you untold hours of stress and emotional turmoil. It also means that you retain some control over the outcome, since mediation involves working with both parties to hammer out a conclusion to the conflict that is mutually acceptable. You don't have to abdicate control of the outcome to a judge. If you are facing such a legal dilemma, seek recommendations of lawyers and other types of professionals who understand the process of mediation and can serve in that capacity. Mediation can save you a great deal of stress, not to mention the financial burden and time involved in taking someone to court.

196. End a Confrontation by Walking Away

An argument by one person is impossible—it always takes two or more people. So what do you think would happen if you just walked away the next time someone became confrontational and tried to start an argument with you? Would that person keep arguing or shouting even if you were in your car driving away? Probably not, but it wouldn't matter anyway because you wouldn't be there to hear the yelling. Confrontations can be over the minute that one person shifts the paradigm. Walk to another office, another room, outside, or elsewhere. The minute you leave the aggressor and retreat to a safe place where he cannot find you, the confrontation is over.

197. Express Your Emotion to Lighten Your Load

Feelings and emotions are almost identical in context. However, there are subtle differences. A feeling is a bodily sensation. If you stub your toe, you feel pain. Emotions are involuntary physical responses to events in life. Examples of an emotional reaction include a blush, a laugh, an increased heart rate, a sudden loss of color, or tears. An emotion may be fleeting or it may remain for days, or even years. The ability to feel enables a person to identify an emotion as something that is either positive or negative. It is when an individual represses an undesirable emotion (such as hidden anger, guilt, or self-hatred) that psychological damage can occur. Acknowledging your emotions and working your way through them will free up your brain.

198. Watch a Funny Movie

Laugh! It really is the best medicine—for both our minds and our bodies. For one thing, a good sense of humor provides needed stress relief. When we laugh at our problems rather than fret over them, they become less serious and thus easier to solve. Humor also improves cognitive function by keeping the mind active and encouraging creative thinking—a vital defense against age—and provides an important emotional catharsis during periods of emotional tension. Laughter helps stimulate the immune system and counters the immunosuppressive effects of stress. So rent a funny movie such as *Annie Hall*, *There's Something about Mary*, *The Blues Brothers*, *Airplane, Mamma Mia, Austin Powers—International Man of Mystery*, or *The Naked Gun*. Or, go to a comedy club or watch a comedic television show such as *The Office* and laugh!

199. Adopt a Pet and Feel Emotionally Lighter and Happier

One of the most consistent findings among the many studies evaluating the beneficial role of pets in our lives is that they provide an important measure of stress relief. Simply petting or playing with our favorite pet, whether it's a dog, cat, hamster, or canary, stimulates the production of calming chemicals within the brain and helps us relax. Watching fish in an aquarium has a similar calming effect. The calming influence of small animals is so effective that many doctors recommend daily pet play as therapy for their patients who are under a lot of stress either at work or at home. Fifteen minutes of tossing a yarn ball to some frolicsome kittens is a wonderful and inexpensive way to shed the stress of a hard day at the office. If you're not a cat person, playing fetch with your dog is equally beneficial. The point is to spend time with your pet, whatever the species, and enjoy its company. Talk to it. Pet it. Scratch it behind the ears. Bask in the glow of the pet-owner bond and feel the anxiety melt away. Even the most stressful day is no match for a puppy that's so happy to see you that its tail is a blur.

chapter ten

Be a True Friend

200. Enjoy a Daily Stroll with Friends

Outings in the fresh air such as walks around the neighborhood just seem more enjoyable when you have one or more friends along. It doesn't have to be a huge chunk of your day—maybe only thirty minutes or an hour. Honor the allotted hour as if it were an important appointment that you have to keep. Friendships need nurturing with quality time and focus. Your body also needs exercise. A daily outing combining a vigorous walk with some stimulating conversation with friends yields a two-fold benefit.

201. Try Out a New Gourmet Recipe on a Neighbor

If you love to cook and try new recipes, share one of your adventurous creations with a neighbor. There's nothing like a homemade dish or special treat to bond people together. Most people understand that cooking takes time, ingredients, and effort on your part. You'll soon discover the other adventurous cooks in the neighborhood. Perhaps they'll begin to invite you to also share samples of their latest food forays. Sharing food is an ancient method of bonding that sometimes results in lifelong friendships.

202. Invite Friends Over for High Tea

A tea party is an opportunity to indulge in an old romantic tradition made famous by the British and French. But you don't have to travel to London or Paris to take afternoon tea with friends. You may be able to find a tea house, hotel, or restaurant that serves a high tea in your own city or town. If not, plan your own tea party. Make it healthier than its traditional counterpart by replacing the white bread sandwiches with a whole-grain bread choice. Offer sliced fruit and strawberries dipped in dark chocolate and fruit tarts with crusts of ground almonds instead of the more traditional heavily sugared sweet cakes and cookies. Whether you host a tea party or do something altogether different, time spent with friends is an important factor in having a higher level of life satisfaction.

203. Take a Friend to the Museum

Love museums but hate going alone? Invite a girlfriend or a guy friend who also loves museums to join you. If the closest museum is miles away, make an afternoon or day of it. Whether it's a museum of modern art, ancient history, or natural science, the exhibits are often visually stimulating (and that can inspire your creativity), and you can learn new information. Plus, you'll be in the stimulating company of a good friend who shares your enthusiasm for museum outings.

204. Make California Rolls with Your Buddies

Cooking together is a great way to strengthen friendships. Invite your buddies over to make California Rolls or other type of sushi. Technically, the word sushi means vinegar rice. California Rolls, one of the easiest and most popular sushi recipes, combines sushi rice with crab meat and bands the moist mound in a paper-thin slice of roasted seaweed. To make California Rolls, which includes avocado and crab meat stuffed in the rice, you'll need a bamboo mat (in which to roll the sushi), a cutting board, a sharp knife, a rice paddle or wooden spoon, and some plastic wrap. Lay out the bamboo mat and cover it with a sheet of plastic wrap. Place on the plastic wrap one sheet of nori (dried, roasted seaweed). Spread about 1 cup of cooked Japanese medium-grain rice over the nori, leaving about a 1-inch border at the edges. Straight across the center of the nori, place chopped cucumber, avocado, and crab. Then, taking one side of the mat and plastic wrap, begin to roll up over the sushi, Roll tightly, then unroll the mat and plastic. Moisten the rolled edge of the nori to seal the roll. Slice the long roll (which is like a rolled cookie dough) into 2-inch pieces and serve on a pretty plate along with condiments such as soy sauce, wasabi (Japanese horseradish), and pickled ginger.

205. Be a Labor Coach for a Pregnant Friend

If you have a friend who is going through a pregnancy alone, offer to be her labor coach. Accompany her to classes such as Lamaze and yoga for pregnant mothers-to-be. Going through a pregnancy can be difficult, with many emotional highs and lows due, in part, to the hormones flooding through the body. In the last trimester, especially, your friend may not feel up to doing many activities. Your friendship during that period will be especially important. Offer to drive her to her appointments, do her grocery shopping, or run errands for her. Whether she is going through the pregnancy alone by choice or because of circumstances of her life, you'll always know your friendship made a positive difference, and you can feel good about that.

206. Be Friendly with Everyone Including the Homeless

Many people refuse to make eye contact with the homeless to avoid the possibility of sparking a conversation that they do not want. While homeless people living on the street suffer hardships that are difficult to imagine and are often treated like society's pariahs, pretending not to see them doesn't void the truth that they are part of society, they are not invisible, and they have dignity, too. Although some may be mentally ill and a minority might even be dangerous, many are ordinary people with few resources and options. Make eye contact, flash a big smile, say hello. Your smile can make a difference and brighten a moment or two for someone others most likely avoid. The look of kindness, compassion, or consideration is more beautiful than an expressionless person who treats others as if they weren't visible.

207. Form a Book Club with a Few Friends

If you are passionate about reading novels and discussing them, find friends, neighbors, and business associates who share your passion. Literature can enrich your life, and the friendships you'll form in a book club increase the size of your social network. Having a strong social network not only contributes to your happiness and well-being, it is an important aspect of having a meaningful life. You'll only need a few people to start your book club. Plan to spend several hours (you can serve appetizers and beverages, if you like) at your home, a local library, or even at a coffee house. The point is to have a designated time and place and to ask everyone to read the same novel and to come prepared to discuss it.

208. Seek Help or Share Your Insights about Beating Addiction

While many Americans are addicted to alcohol, prescription or illegal drugs, gambling, or have other types of addiction, there are also many who are recovering addicts and who receive support in staying sober from Alcoholics Anonymous or Narcotics Anonymous organizations. Addiction recovery necessarily is an ongoing process. The first step is for the individual to admit he or she has a problem. Since alcoholism requires treatment by professionals who understand how the process of becoming addicted takes hold in the brain as well as the best methods for breaking the cycle, support for the addicted individual becomes paramount. If you are addicted, seek help so you can feel better and again have a meaningful life. If you are someone who has already recovered, attend an AA meeting and offer to tell your personal story and insights about beating the addiction. Help others reclaim their lives.

209. Allow a Friend to Grow and Change

Friends who deeply care about each other permit their friends (and their friendships) to grow, change, and evolve. If your friend is seeking some answers to a life issue and it means that she is growing in a new direction that challenges some of your beliefs, do you become confrontational? For example, say that you and your friend have always shared a strong belief that husbands and wives must stay together for the sake of their children regardless of the family dynamics. But your friend and her husband have hit a long, rough patch and she tells you she is filing for divorce. Resist the temptation to protest and argue your position. Instead, be loving and supportive. If she wants to talk, be an active listener. Try not to influence her with your own biases, and be the friend you would want her to be for you if your roles were reversed.

210. Help a Friend Who Is Feeling Rejected

Criticism, even if it's well intentioned, can feel like rejection. If you have a friend who is feeling down because a boss, coworker, a spouse, a partner, or someone else made a critical remark, remind your friend to put it into perspective. The criticism, although directed at the individual, may not have been about that person, but about a task or obligation needing completion against a deadline. It could have come about because a superior was criticized and she just took it out on your friend. Whatever the reason, the result was the same. Share with your friend a personal story of a time when that happened to you, too. Help your friend make sense of it. A true friend tries to understand and help a friend in need.

211. Support a Friend in Starting a Green Project or Business

If you have a friend who wants to grow heirloom, organic vegetables for local restaurants but needs various types of assistance, why not wholeheartedly support him? Whether you are asked to pull weeds, fill crates, do planting, deliver produce, work on the clerical side, or lend monetary assistance, do what you can and give what you are able. Whenever anyone is doing something good for the environment and the effort benefits other people, it's a venture worth supporting. And since supporting the cause means you will be also strengthening your friendship, it's easy to see how getting involved could nurture both your own spirit and body.

212. Make New Friends at Sponsored Events

Many foundations use some form of group exercise in a concerted effort to raise money and awareness for their causes. You could get involved in playing in a charity golf tournament, ride in the annual cycling event sponsored by the Leukemia and Lymphoma Foundation, or walk for the American Heart Association or the American Cancer Society. You will be working out while making new friends with some kindred spirits. Expanding your social network and shared experience can increase your life's purpose, meaning, and enjoyment—always a good thing.

213. Back Off When Your Friend Requests It

Inevitably, in many close friendships, a time comes when you have to go against your inclination to be helpful and instead just back off. For example, your best friend, who has long-standing issues with certain members of his family and who has broken off all contact with them, has asked you not to interfere or to bring his family up in conversations. Despite your desire to encourage him to reestablish contact and restart a dialogue with his family, don't. Although your intention is well meaning, the best thing you can do is to honor your friendship and respect his wishes.

214. Help Your Friend Raise Money for College

If you have a friend starting or returning to college, offer to set aside some time to help her brainstorm ways to raise the necessary money. Finding scholarships, educational grants, and other sources of money can be daunting. Helping her could inspire you to return to college as well to complete your own degree or earn another. You already know that the process of learning new information keeps your brain young.

215. Offer to Be a Guardian for Your Friend's Children

Parents are wise to decide upon someone to care for all their children under the age of eighteen in the event that they become incapacitated or otherwise unable to care for them and to spell out their choice in a legal document. Have a heart-to-heart talk with your closest friend about his choice for who would raise his children if he could not. Offer to raise his children in the unlikely event that becomes necessary and only if that option feels right to you. Encourage him to seek the help of a lawyer and establish his wishes in a legal document such as a living will, a trust, or a notarized letter.

216. Stay in Touch with Old Friends

If you have noticed that through the decades the company you keep changes, you are not alone. In fact, it's fairly common as we grow older to form new and different groups of friends. Some people manage to have the same friends throughout their lives, while others don't. When you are young, you might form many friendships but, most likely, few of them will last over a lifetime. When people marry, have families, and move away from where they grew up or attended college, friendships are often the casualties of that change. Through the instability of life, hold on to your friendships for the support and anchoring they provide. Stay in contact with those who move and keep track of old friends. A strong social network (especially with old friends) becomes increasingly important as you age.

217. Support a Friend Going Through a Legal Process

Nothing can be as disempowering as having to go through a legal process alone, especially if you don't understand the steps in the process or are intimidated by court proceedings. Whether your friend is dealing with a do-it-yourself divorce or is working with an attorney to contest a contractual dispute or adopting a child, be encouraging and supportive as she fills out paperwork or prepares for interviews, or attends court proceedings. Be a good listener, give your insights only when asked, and offer hugs when they are needed.

218. Share Knowledge of Healing Herbs with a Friend

If you have always loved to keep a garden with herbs for healing, share your knowledge with a friend. Through history, women have been natural healers, using fresh and dried herbs and wholesome fruits and vegetables to make ointments, oils, tinctures, teas, and poultices. When it comes to the healing arts, two minds working together could be better than one working alone. Imagine how much fun it will be to share ideas with your friend and to pour over seed catalogues, exchange herbal remedies, and discuss the healing properties of the various herbs that you both can grow in your pots or gardens. In addition, through the body of knowledge you share, you may be able to help each other to stave off illnesses and stay healthy and strong over your lifetimes.

219. Give a Party for Charity

Invite friends and family to join you for a different kind of party that celebrates friendship and loving family connections. Or, for a twist on the usual, make your next dinner or cocktail gathering a party with a purpose. Put out decorative boxes for donations and theme the event around the charity that you're collecting for. For help choosing a worthy organization to donate to, visit *www.charitywatch.org* or *www.charitynavigator.org*.

chapter eleven

Protect Yourself Against Age-Related Diseases

220. Make a Daily Commitment to Be Healthy

If you're like many people who allow years to pass before they decide that good health should be a priority, take heart. It's never too late to make that commitment to exercise regularly, initiate lifestyle changes, and eat more nutritious foods. However, the earlier you start, the bigger the payoff. You could add years to your lifespan and improve the way you look and feel with just a few modifications to your current lifestyle. A strong, fit, toned, healthy, beautiful body is, in fact, the product of a healthy lifestyle. Make a promise to yourself every day to commit your lifestyle and food choices to those that ensure optimum health and reduce your risk for acquiring age-related diseases.

221. Eat Egg Yolks for Your Eyesight

Eggs and green leafy vegetables such as kale and spinach are all high in lutein, but yellow egg yolks are considered one of the best sources because they are easily available and absorbed better by the body than other sources of lutein. Lutein, an antioxidant that your body cannot make, protects the underlying eye tissues from phototoxic damage by filtering out ultraviolet light in sunshine, and blocking harmful free radicals in the eye. This damage may be a factor in cataracts and age-related macular degeneration (ARMD), the leading cause of blindness in the United States. Increasing foods rich in lutein may decrease the risk of developing advanced or exudative ARMD, the most visually disabling form of macular degeneration among older people. Experts believe antioxidant nutrients, including lutein, not only may help to prevent eye diseases, but may help prevent further deterioration of existing conditions. Try scrambling an egg for breakfast. One large yolk is only about 59 calories and is a major source of vitamins A, D, K, and E, minerals, and also cholesterol, while the white (or albumen) is only about 100 calories and contains protein but no fat.

222. Discover What You Can Do to Avoid Alzheimer's

Approximately 4 million Americans are believed to have Alzheimer's disease, 90 percent of them over age sixty. The brains of Alzheimer's patients contain distinctive, abnormally shaped proteins known as tangles and plaques. Tangles are long, silk-like tendrils found inside neurons. Plaques are clumps of silk-like fibers that typically form outside the neurons in adjacent brain tissue. The areas most commonly afflicted by tangles and plaques are related to memory. In the 1980s, researchers found that a compound in plaques, known as amyloid protein, may actually be poisonous to brain cells. A protein called tau may be responsible for the telltale tangles found in the brains of Alzheimer's patients. In healthy brains, tau gives neurons structural support. Take the time to research Alzheimer's and other forms of dementia and learn what you might do to reduce your risk factors for developing any type of dementia.

223. Walk Away from Heart Attack Risk

Regular physical activity keeps our muscles toned and strong, helps us maintain our ideal weight by burning calories, maintains bone strength and density, and improves and maintains heart and lung function. Exercise also builds stamina, improves flexibility, boosts our immune system, makes sex more fun, reduces our risk of cancer, improves our reflexes, lowers stress, and benefits our overall physical and mental health. In addition, exercise helps keep our metabolism functioning at maximum capacity, which becomes increasingly important as we age and find it increasingly difficult to process fatty acids. This, in turn, affects almost all of the body's systems, diminishing immune response and increasing our risk of atherosclerotic disease. Simply taking a thirty-minute walk every day can reduce your risk of heart attack after just five months, doctors report.

224. Thwart the Onset of Osteoporosis

Bone is an active tissue that is constantly undergoing "remodeling" that involves resorption (old bone is removed) and formation (new bone is formed). The rate of remodeling in children can be as high as 50 percent per year compared to about 5 percent in adults. Until the age of 30 or so, we build and store bone efficiently. Then, as part of the aging process, bones begin to break down faster than new bone can be formed. If bone calcium stores are not sufficient, as the aging process takes over, the risk of osteoporosis increases. If you are at risk for developing osteoporosis, talk with your doctor about what you can do. Often physicians recommend changes in nutrition, exercise, and lifestyle. You may want to increase your intake of calcium and vitamin D (since vitamin D helps the absorption of calcium) and also start some weight-bearing exercise such as walking, climbing stairs, or jogging because bones, like muscles, can respond to exercise.

225. Stave Off Colon Cancer

Colon cancer is one of the most common cancers in the Western world. Research has shown that colon cancer incidence rates are inversely proportional to calcium intake—as intakes go up, cancer rates go down. One study indicates that most cases of colon cancer may be prevented with regular calcium intake for men and women of around 1,800 milligrams and 1,000 milligrams per 1,000 calories per day, respectively, along with 800 IUs of vitamin D per day. Researchers suspect that calcium may prevent polyp formation by binding to carcinogens and thereby inhibiting abnormal cell growth.

226. See Trans Fat as a Silent Killer

Trans fat is an artificial fat produced when liquid vegetable oil is treated with heat, chemicals, and hydrogen to transform it into a product that is semisolid at room temperature. The fat is used instead of animal fats like butter or lard because it is easier to work with, doesn't become rancid, and can be used over and over again without breaking down or burning. Fats are notoriously volatile, become rancid quickly, are difficult to store, and can be very expensive. So when hydrogenated fat was invented it seemed like a quick and easy answer for food processors. But, the truth is that trans fat is one of the few food ingredients that is truly bad for you. Avoid it like you would the plague if you want to maintain good cardiovascular health and lower the risk of heart attack and stroke.

227. Give Your Brain Good Fats

Each nerve cell in the brain is surrounded by a protective cell membrane. Receptors for many brain neurotransmitters are found on the membrane. This membrane is composed mostly of different types of fats, which include phosphatidylcholine (PC), also called lecithin; phosphatidylserine (PS); and phosphatidylethanolamine (PE). The function of the nerve cells and the neurotransmitters is highly dependent on the quality of fats that make up the cell membrane and therefore highly dependent on the type of fats and oils in your diet. The makeup of a cell membrane is always in a state of transition; it is constantly influenced by diet, stress, and the immune system. The bottom line: Your brain needs "good fats" like omega-3 fats, found in nuts, avocados and extra-virgin olive oil.

228. Know Your Homocysteine Levels

In 1969, elevated levels of an amino acid called homocysteine were found in the urine of patients with heart disease. Homocysteine is a normal by-product of protein digestion. If it occurs in elevated amounts it can cause cholesterol to change into an "oxidized," or rancid, form, which goes on to damage blood vessels. In the *New England Journal of Medicine* on February 14, 2002, the Boston University Medical Center reported on an eight-year study. In 1,092 patients, an increase in plasma homocysteine level of 5 μmol/liter increased the risk of Alzheimer's disease by 40 percent. The highest levels doubled the risk. If various B vitamins (B12, B6, and folic acid) are deficient in your diet, homocysteine builds up. Be aware that heart disease often correlates to brain dysfunction. If homocysteine is a marker for risk to cardiovascular health, better keep an eye on it.

229. See Coffee as a Drug and Use It in Moderation

According to the National Coffee Association, 80 percent of Americans drink coffee, and occasional coffee consumption rose 6 percent in the last year. At the same time, panic and other anxiety disorders have become the most common mental illnesses in the United States. Professionals agree that when caffeine overlaps with these disorders, the result can be trouble. Roland Griffiths, Ph.D., a professor in the Departments of Psychiatry and Neuroscience at the Johns Hopkins University School of Medicine states, "Caffeine is the most widely used mood-altering drug in the world. People often see coffee, tea, and soft drinks simply as beverages rather than vehicles for a psychoactive drug. But caffeine can exacerbate anxiety and panic disorders. Use it in moderation. As you age and your body necessarily experiences lots of changes, resist the temptation to drink lots of coffee for the caffeine boost it gives. Too much can cause palpitations and irritability."

230. Boost Metabolism to Keep Away Age-Related Brain Problems

All activity in the body occurs through a process called metabolism in which cells break down chemicals and nutrients to generate energy and form new molecules like proteins. Efficient metabolism requires blood loaded with oxygen, glucose, and nutrients. Enzymes are the molecules that make metabolism happen, and nutrients are vitamins and minerals that act as essential co-enzymes. When a nutrient is deficient in the body, certain metabolic functions are impeded and symptoms of disease can arise. Eat a healthy diet, exercise, and keep your body in top running form, and it may just help stave off age-related brain diseases.

231. Get Enough Sleep to Ward Off Age-Related Accidents

Your body, including your brain, actually mends and maintains itself when you rest and sleep. Getting enough sleep as you grow older helps you stay safe; being sleep-deprived increases the likelihood of having accidents and making mistakes. As you reach your forties and fifties, most likely you'll notice that your eyesight isn't what it once was. Sleep won't help your eyesight, but it may enable your brain to function better and be more alert to what you see. Likewise, as you age, it's important to remember that your reflexes also might not respond as quickly as when you were in your teens or early twenties. Give your brain the rest it needs to stay sharp so that when you need to take quick action in response to something you see, like a car stopped ahead of you in traffic because of dense fog, you are able to react in time to ensure your safety.

232. Learn about the Link Between Sugar Intake and Age-Related Disease

Sugars are simple carbohydrates that the body uses as a source of energy. During digestion, all carbohydrates break down into sugar, or blood glucose. They are also stored in the muscles and liver as glycogen. Some sugars occur naturally, but sugar is often added in food processing or preparation. Most foods containing added sugars provide calories but little else. The body cannot tell the difference between naturally occurring sugar and added sugar. Diabetes, which can accelerate the aging process, occurs when your body cannot properly regulate its blood sugar. New research suggests that a low-carbohydrate diet as well as a daily cup of coffee might lower the risk for developing certain types of diabetes, however; research is ongoing.

233. Mix an Anti-Aging Tonic

A folk remedy of high and pure repute, apple cider vinegar, was mentioned by the Greek physician Hippocrates as a healing elixir and energizing tonic. His recommendation to take one to two teaspoons of raw apple cider vinegar and one to two teaspoons raw honey mixed in eight ounces of water has been passed down over thousands of years right to the present day, where it is touted by many alternative healers as being beneficial for all parts of the body. Apple cider vinegar is made from freshly pressed apple juice that is first fermented into a hard apple cider and then fermented once again into apple cider vinegar. This process allows for the vinegar to retain all the nutritional value of the apples, and provides the added benefit of powerful enzymes created during the fermentation process.

234. Monitor Your Cholesterol Values and Know What They Mean

If you have a cholesterol reading over 240 milligrams per decilitre or you have risk factors such as heart disease along with cholesterol readings over 200 milligrams per decilitre, your doctor will probably prescribe a cholesterol-lowering medication in combination with a healthy low-fat diet and exercise. Your doctor should periodically test your blood cholesterol levels to check on your progress. Take action as necessary to keep your cholesterol levels appropriate for your age.

235. Avoid Risks Associated with Brain Attack (Stroke)

Brain attack, cerebrovascular accident (CVA), and stroke all refer to a rapid loss of brain function brought on by some kind of change in its blood supply, whether that change has been caused by a clot, a rupture and bleed, blockage, interruption of blood flow due to heart failure, or loss of the blood supply because of illicit drug use, for example. Currently, stroke is the third leading cause of death in America. People age fifty-five and older are at highest risk because for each decade of life past age fifty-five, the incidence of stroke more than doubles. Some of the risk factors that you may be able to change or modify, thus reducing the risk of stroke, include high blood pressure, high cholesterol levels, smoking, unhealthy diet, obesity, alcohol use, drug use, and lack of physical activity.

236. Take Care of Your Kidneys

Kidneys filter your blood, removing wastes and any extra water. As you age, your kidneys may experience age-related changes as well. The kidneys continue to function normally unless they become stressed. Diabetes mellitus and high blood pressure are two age-related diseases that can stress and impair kidney function. Kidney disease can also trigger hypertension. A blood clot to the lung or a myocardial infarction can bring about shutdown in kidney function. Salt and water intake can also affect the kidneys as they age. Kidneys won't be as good holding water volume as you get older. Thus, you may need to get up in the middle of the night to urinate. Protect your kidneys by keeping your insulin and blood sugars at a normal, healthy level, eating small to moderate amounts of protein (instead of a high-protein diet that puts more work on the kidneys), and moderate amounts of non-starchy veggies. Avoid nonsteroidal anti-inflammatory drugs and if you smoke, stop.

237. Switch from Butter to Cholesterol-Lowering Margarines

Various margarines on the market today are low in both saturated fats and trans fatty acids. Trans fatty acids are created through the process of hydrogenation. They can increase LDL cholesterol and lower HDL. Many of these margarines are called "spreads" because they are less than 80 percent oil. The more solid a margarine is, the more saturated fat and trans fat they contain. When looking for margarine spreads, look for a margarine spread with no more than 30 percent fat from saturated plus trans fat. Less than 20 percent is even better. Also, look for a word such as trans-free, which means the spread has no more than half a gram of trans fat per serving. But be sure they are not replacing trans fats with saturated fats. These new margarine spreads are not a magic bullet to lowering cholesterol, but in moderation they can be part of your heart-healthy lifestyle.

238. Stabilize Mood Swings to Thwart Cognitive Impairment

Preliminary but exciting new research suggests that omega-3 fatty acids may help decrease symptoms of bipolar disorder (or manic depression). Researchers at Harvard University suggest that omega-3 fats may interfere with the brain signals that trigger the characteristic mood swings seen with bipolar disorder. Interestingly, the investigators reported unusually high patient interest and acceptance of omega-3 fatty acids as mood stabilizers. The supplements were viewed as "natural" compounds with few side effects. If these findings hold true in future studies, omega-3 fatty acids may have implications for treating other psychiatric disorders such as depression and schizophrenia. Try taking at least ten grams of fish oil a day to see if it helps with mood stabilization. If you have been diagnosed as bipolar, do not substitute fish oil for your medication. An article published in *Bipolar Disorders* and written by Dr. Carrie Bearden at the University of Pennsylvania explores the link between neuropsychological deficits and the length of time patients had suffered bipolar illness. It concludes that wild mood swings possibly damage the brain's memory and learning systems. The disorder also has been linked to diabetes, migraines, and hypothyroidism. If you are a bipolar sufferer, talk to your doctor about stabilizing severe mood swings.

239. Protect Your Hearing as You Age

Hearing tends to peak at puberty, and gradually declines after that, though many baby boomers no doubt hastened their hearing loss with too much loud music when they were younger. In fact, hearing experts anticipate a dramatic increase in hearing problems among boomers fifty and younger, due to a lack of precautions during their teens, twenties, and thirties. Generally speaking, sensitivity to the higher tones is the first to go, particularly among men. Nutrition, environment, occupation, and other factors can also play a role in hearing loss as we age. Take care of your hearing and understand the factors that can bring about hearing loss, such as listening to the radio with the volume cranked up or attending a concert and sitting or standing near loud speakers.

240. Don't Give Up Activities That Give You Pleasure

Slowing down as you age is one thing. But so many people reach the age of retirement and then just stop doing things, such as shopping with friends, staying active, engaging their brains in the pursuit of lifelong learning, or attending cultural events. For some, it's as if they were just waiting for the end. Live every day to its fullest, as if it were the last. Have fun. For the heck of it, visualize your last day. Are you dressed in your black cocktail mini with a martini glass in one hand and the hand of your dance partner in the other? So you slip on that banana peel. At least you went out doing something you loved with someone whose company you enjoyed, and wearing a nifty little number that made you look and feel beautiful. The point is that life isn't over until it's over.

241. Work to Lower Your LDL and Raise Your HDL

The less LDL (bad cholesterol) you have and the more HDL (good cholesterol) you have, the lower your risk for heart disease. When it comes to trying to lower your LDL, food choices are key. A combination of a diet low in saturated fat and cholesterol, regular physical activity, and a healthy weight can help you lower your total cholesterol as well as raise your HDL, lower your LDL, and lower your triglycerides. It is important to focus on your cholesterol intake as well as your saturated fat intake, which often occur together in foods. Cholesterol and most saturated fats come *only* from animal foods. Even though some foods of plant origin are high in fat or saturated fat, all plant foods are cholesterol-free. Nuts, for example, are high in fat—mostly unsaturated fat—but are cholesterol-free.

chapter twelve

Give Your Life Meaning Through Good Works

242. Write Your Vision for a Purposeful Life

Ponder the question: Where do I want to go in my life and what do I want to do that will give my life purpose and meaning and will also give me satisfaction? What endeavor, project, or cause might I work on that would leave me feeling renewed, regenerated, and inspired? Then, after you visualize a snapshot of your future just as you want it to be, write what you have envisioned. Think about how you would adjust or tweak your snapshot in order to get more clarity. Where are you in the world? What is your work? What are you doing? Are you alone or with others? Who is with you? How much money do you have? Are you happy? Do you like the person you see in that snapshot?

243. Aspire to Excellence in Your Volunteer Work

Choose to do some volunteer work such as spearheading a food or clothing drive, setting up a community outreach program for shut-ins, or working a crisis hotline phone bank. Aspire to excellence in each task you do. Whether you are passing cartons of milk at snack time at a local school for underprivileged children, coordinating an art show for a group of at-risk teens, or playing piano at a senior center on Sunday afternoons, put care, consideration, focus, style, and vitality into what you do. Performing your work well demonstrates your level of commitment to others.

244. Buy a Subway Pass for Someone Who Can't Afford It

When you notice someone who doesn't have enough money to purchase a ticket or a pass for the subway, consider purchasing it for him. Performing a spontaneous, selfless act of kindness generates good karma for you while helping the other guy. You don't know what that person's circumstances of life are like. Your simple act of generosity could brighten the day of someone whose life may have more lack than abundance or misery than happiness. Performing such charitable acts and helping others can give your own life more meaning and purpose.

245. Join Global Partners to Fight Tobacco-Related Illness and Death

One in five deaths in the United States is caused by tobacco use, according to the American Cancer Society. Even though it is well known that cigarettes, chewing tobacco, and snuff are addictive, tobacco use among adolescents is on the rise. Tobacco use can cause heart disease, cancer, and lung disease such as emphysema. While the tobacco industry profits greatly from the global markets for its product, groups all over the world are joining together to fight what they consider the global epidemic of tobacco-related illness and death. Expand your network of contacts in the world while working for a cause that resonates with your beliefs.

246. Register to Be a Bone Marrow Donor

A bone marrow transplant is a life-saving treatment for some people with leukemia, certain genetic disorders, or immune disease. Such a treatment option necessarily requires that donors be closely matched to the recipient or individual needing the transplant. The National Marrow Donor (NMD) program naturally looks to family members first and then to people on its registry. That's why it needs a large pool of people willing to be listed in its registry as potential donors. Since anesthesia is used on the donor, there is generally no pain with the extraction procedure. Only liquid marrow is removed, no bone is taken. Afterward the donor may feel low-back pain for a few days. Get the facts at *www.marrow.org*.

247. Spearhead a Gift Drive for a Children's Shelter

Check with a local children's shelter to see what its gifting policy and needs are for its young residents. You don't have to wait until the December holiday season to consider a gift drive. Birthdays occur in all seasons. Books are always welcome for readers of all levels. If you decide you want to help out a local children's shelter, find out first the ages of the children and get a recommendation for age-appropriate gifts and books. Then do whatever you feel inspired to do to make a birthday or holiday special for a child in a shelter. Your effort can make a huge difference in the life of a child experiencing a transition in her life.

248. Be a Foster Parent

Foster parents provide safe, stable, and supportive environments for children who have been removed temporarily from their families. Being a foster parent can be a life-changing experience. As a foster parent you serve as a member of a team working with the birth family to enable the child in your care to reunite at some point with his birth family. In the event the child cannot return to the birth family, you may consider adopting that child to provide him with a permanent home.

249. Demonstrate a Recycle Mindset for Others

Establish a company-wide recycling program if your company doesn't already have such a program in place. Take your concerns to your supervisor or boss and work with the operations department to get quotes from local recycling plants. Obtain bids from those with the best deals. Recycling benefits your company, community, and the planet. Do your part to demonstrate the importance of recycling paper, boxes, ink cartridges, water bottles, soda cans, and all other "waste" products produced at your place of work. By showing how to think like a habitual recycler, you might just start a recycling culture that could expand outward into your community, county, and beyond.

250. Help an Entrepreneur in the Developing World

Nothing changes a life more than learning to be self-sufficient and having your own company or idea for making money. If you want to make a donation and know that it's making a very specific difference, look into an organization like the Foundation for International Community Assistance at *www.villagebanking.org*. These companies allow you to make a loan to an entrepreneur in the developing world and learn the specific use of the money. Evaluate that option to see if it feels right to you and if it gives you some sense of purpose.

251. Make an Offering to Your House of Worship's Global Mission

Your offering enables your house of worship to alleviate hunger and to serve impoverished and sick people in America and abroad. Find out what members of your faith are doing through global outreach to make the world a better place. Gather up your loose change and make a donation. Or you can make a cross-religion donation and give money to another religion's charitable efforts.

252. Invest in Socially Responsible Funds

Learn about investing and ways to grow your money while staying true to your sense of the social good. Talk with friends who like investing and invite them to join you in putting your discretionary income into socially responsible investing. Companies like Equal Exchange are letting you put your saved money to good use, and get it back! Visit *www.equalexchange.com/eecd* for more information. To learn more about socially responsible investing including a very detailed analysis of various options, visit *www.socialfunds.com.*

253. Host a Benefit

People love gathering together over worthy causes, and it makes the act of donating more sociable. If you can't attend or organize one on your own, consider volunteering for a benefit. With people like you volunteering to serve food, the overhead costs are lowered and more of the proceeds can go directly to the organization.

254. Save a Quarter Every Day

While it might be hard to budget large donations to charitable organizations, consider setting aside a quarter a day in a hunger fund. Once the quarters start to pile up, take them to the bank and then write out a check (see *www.bread.org* for donating to hunger organizations).

255. Hold a Yard Sale

Why sell old junk just to buy new junk? Advertise your yard sale by proclaiming that "all proceeds benefit orphans displaced by the tsunami." Plus, people are less likely to haggle over prices if they know that their money is going to support a worthy cause!

256. Organize a Bake Sale

You can have a bake sale in your local school or other meeting place. Try making it themed with the charity you're raising funds for. For example, make sugar cookies and cut them into the shape of Africa if you're fundraising for AIDS in Africa.

257. Meet People with the Same Political Beliefs as You

Link up with other like-minded people. Make an effort to meet other politically active people by attending political rallies, working with charitable fundraisers, and joining environmental groups for hikes, bird watching, or biking trips. When you join communities of like-minded people, you have more power to effect change, get laws enacted, and do good works.

258. Join the Effort to Find a Cure for an Incurable Disease

There are many from which to choose, including HIV/AIDS, many types of cancer, multiple sclerosis, autism, cystic fibrosis, polio, and Tay-Sachs, to mention a few. Choose a disease, research how you can help, and get involved. Now make that cause your mission. Get off the couch, out of the house, and make your life count in the effort to save someone else's life. Doing so will give meaning and purpose to your own life, and that, as you already know, translates to higher life satisfaction and longevity.

259. Donate Your Old Eyeglasses

You're not using them anymore and someone who needs eyeglasses would appreciate receiving them. An organization called Unite for Sight can get your old eyeglasses to people who need them. Find out more at *www.uniteforsight.org*. Americans toss out approximately 4 million eyeglasses each year—eyewear that could benefit people in the developing world with vision loss. What you may be taking for granted, being able to purchase a good pair of glasses, could be a luxury to someone who either can't afford them or doesn't have access to vision or medical care personnel.

260. Get in Shape for a Worthwhile Cause

Earn money for medical research teams and exercise at the same time by participating in a charity walk. Join forces with the Leukemia Foundation for a Cure or the Fight against Breast Cancer or the American Heart Association and walk to raise money for medical research. You'll be working that beautiful body of yours for an admirable and worthwhile purpose.

261. Get Involved in a Mental Health Charity

Hollywood celebrities sometimes use the power of their fame to aid charitable causes. For example, Hugh Laurie, lead actor on the television series *House* and a sometime sufferer of clinical depression, is just one celebrity involved in charitable work benefiting The National Alliance on Mental Illness. That charitable organization works to improve life quality for people with mental illness as well as research preventative methods and to find cures. You don't have to be a celebrity to make a difference in the life of someone who suffers from mental illness. But you do have to get involved. Many mental health charities are listed on the Internet. Find one you'd like to work with and make that call.

chapter thirteen

Indulge in Frequent Loving Sex

262. Put Yourself in the Mood

When you want to play between the sheets, give yourself time to unwind from your workday and shift into a sexy mood. Ask your spouse to make you a cocktail or pour you a glass of wine and put on some romantic music. Perhaps you have time for a soothing bath, refreshing shower, or a few yoga stretches. Invite your spouse to join you. After bathing, you could slip into silky, sexy underwear, lounging clothes, or a nightie. Tease your partner into a playful pillow fight or a wrestling match. When you are having fun and drawing close, it's easier to feel romantic.

263. Try a Sexy Herb from Peru

The Peruvian herb maca, with over 1,000 years of safe use behind it, is proven to enhance libido and sexual function, according to Chris Kilham in *Better Nutrition* (September 1999). He says that maca, which is consumed throughout Peru, has achieved status as a bona fide aphrodisiac. Tests conducted on maca reveal no toxicity and a complete absence of adverse pharmacologic effects. Kilham writes: "For every health need, nature offers a solution, usually in the form of a safe, healthful plant. Maca may well provide tough competition for Viagra, and become a popular aphrodisiac—for men and women alike—in the United States." Take Maca either in capsule or powder form. Since the powder form is somewhat bitter, you may want to take it in a gelatinized form, which is less bitter and nuttier tasting. The powder form can be sprinkled on foods after first mixing it with a hot or cold liquid. A quarter teaspoon to one teaspoonful twice each day is considered a fairly standard dose. Learn more at *www.macadata.com/taking.php.*

264. Be a Sex Goddess for Your Spouse

Sometimes it's cool to get wild and crazy. For your husband's birthday, for example, keep the guest list really short, say, just the two of you. Show him a totally different side of your personality. You don't have to look like the Playmate of the Year, but it might be fun for both of you if you could slip into a sexy little outfit that puts a little sizzle and sense of expectation in the air. If you want to go really loco, cook him a gourmet meal, set the table for two, and then forgo clothes for an apron-only, jewelry and stilettos look. Discover how exciting a birthday party can be.

265. Sip an Aphrodisiac Tea

Sometimes depression or anxiety makes happy sexual functioning difficult. This may be because your energy is too low, or it may be connected with a hormone imbalance. Damiana stimulates both the nervous and hormonal systems, containing constituents that convert to hormones in the body. Vervain releases tension and stress and was traditionally used as an aphrodisiac. Wild oats and ginger are both stimulating, as well. Ginger is even said to fire the blood. Make an herbal tea with a teaspoon of dried damiana and a teaspoon of dried vervain in a pot with two and a half cups of boiling water. Steep for ten minutes. Strain and flavor with licorice, ginger, or honey. Drink two cups a day. This will restore energy of all kinds.

266. Share Some Sexy Foods Such as Raw Oysters

Raw oysters may stand supreme in the sexy food category as an age-old aphrodisiac. They are high in zinc, which is believed to increase male sperm and testosterone production. Scientists believe that testosterone plays a more major role in sex drive and arousal for both men and women than estrogen alone. Lemon juice drizzled over the oysters helps brighten their flavor. Other foods touted as aphrodisiacs through the centuries include eggs, caviar, avocado, figs, clams, mussels, basil, foie gras, asparagus, bananas, almonds, and chocolate. Get imaginative about making a meal out of sexy foods and do your own research into whether or not they are a factor in sexual arousal.

267. Play a Role-Reversal Game

Play nurse to his doctor, waitress to his chef, or law student to his honor, the judge. Have fun reversing your roles. Keep the playful attitude going full throttle to sexually charge your togetherness. Try a little soft bondage, but only if neither of you have issues about that kind of foreplay. Keep it light and sexy and playful and see what develops. Psychologists say playing and having fun together deepens your feelings toward each other.

268. Read His Palm to Ignite His Passion

Playfully read his palm. While sensuously tracing the lines of his hands, tell him things like, "This is the hand of a very passionate man," or "Someone is about to show you how much passion she feels for you," or "a hot, passionate romp is in your immediate future." That will undoubtedly inspire him to ask how immediate. You can either answer him by saying "now" or have fun with it, stretching out the palm reading session to playfully tease and titillate through your sexy banter.

269. Take a Steamy Shower Together

If your spouse tends to get in the shower before you in the morning, slip out of bed and step into the shower with her. Soap her back, moving your hands slowly and sensuously over her shoulders and back. Guide your soapy palms down both her arms. Momentarily intertwine your fingers with hers. Move closer so that your body touches hers. A steamy, sexy shower together is a terrific way to get going in the morning and to feel great all day.

270. Pack a Picnic Supper to Eat at Sunset

Sunsets are beautiful and romantic, made more so when you are sharing a meal in the company of someone you love. In a picnic basket, pack a small supper along with a bottle of wine or sparkling apple cider to share with your lover while watching the sunset from a high hill, an empty field, your backyard, a local park, at a lake's edge, or in some isolated cove along a beach. In that magical hour between daylight and twilight, draw close, nibble on his neck, and whisper sweet words of love. Shaking up your couple's routine could have wonderful consequences.

271. Give Your Lover an Erotic-Style Massage

For a variant of traditional massage, try body against body, skin-to-skin. Not only is it sensuous, it can stimulate sexy feelings in both of you. Rub fragrant massage oil onto your body and then begin gently massaging your partner. Move on top of your partner, gently positioning your chest and tummy against hers. Now lightly lift yourself so as to move your torso against her chest, making long strokes. Try it with your lower body, abdomen, hips, and thighs against hers.

272. Watch a Documentary Together about the World's Oldest Profession

If you don't discover some sexy secrets, you'll at least learn a little historical information because historical documentaries nearly always provide context. Plus, you can bet that you and your partner will have plenty to talk about during and after the show. Some guys and ladies, too, become stimulated with sex talk and images, so think about watching it in your room, from the comfort of your own bed. Don't be surprised if afterward, sleep is the last thing on your mind.

273. Have Great Sex . . . Regularly

Sex not only feels good, it's good for you. Regular sexual activity is good for your brain, your mood, pain relief, and memory. Having an orgasm decreases pain activity by 50 percent. Having sex three times a week decreases heart attack and stroke by 50 percent. Regular sexual activity ultimately can help you live longer. This isn't just theory; it's clinical fact. A Duke University longitudinal study on aging found a strong correlation between the frequency and enjoyment of sexual intercourse and longevity. And a more recent British study had the same result, noting lower overall rates of mortality among men who have sex far more frequently than the once-a-week national average. Bottom line: Men and women who have frequent, loving sex tend to live longer than those who don't.

274. Let Orgasms Boost Your Self-Esteem

Orgasms are good on so many levels, obviously. Sex, in general, is stimulated by and stimulates the right hemisphere of your brain, the one associated with creativity, music, social skills, spirituality, and pleasure. During orgasm, blood flows into the right prefrontal cortex, creating that fabulous sense of release and gratification. Orgasms also stimulate deep emotional parts of the brain and thus provide a calming influence. Those who have orgasms experience less depression than those who do not. According to Werner Habermehl, a German sex researcher, the more sex you have, the smarter you become. He credits the stimulation of adrenaline and cortisol during lovemaking, plus the bonus surge of serotonin and endorphins that follows orgasm. Regular orgasms ultimately lead to a boost in self-esteem.

275. Try the "Pair of Tongs" Kama Sutra Position

Ever tire of having sex the same way? If you experiment imaginatively before, during, and after sex, you can get in plenty of stretches and a decent cardio workout. Of course, you will also stimulate the flow of those pleasurable and dreamy endorphins that makes sex so enjoyable. If you can't think of any new ways to turn on, tantalize, and titillate your partner, consider the vast world of positions found in tantric yoga practice. Read the Kama Sutra to find out variations on the best-known positions and interesting new positions such as the "Twining Position" or the "The Circle" and the "Pair of Tongs." Visit your local bookstore or Amazon.com for books that can provide "positional" insights. It just may put the sizzle back into your sexual relationship.

276. Avoid Fault Finding

If you think your significant other has faults, consider the possibility that you do, too. Everyone has faults, but that doesn't mean you are stuck with yours. Pick one you would like to change or eliminate. Take time to do a little self-examination with complete honesty. Do you complain about his seemingly voracious sexual appetite when you are tired or his lack of it when you are in the mood? Are you given to sniping and grousing because he doesn't spend enough time on foreplay? Do you have a quick temper and a short fuse that is robbing your relationship of intimacy? Do you procrastinate and avoid talking about your bedroom issues until they snowball out of control? Or, are you still blaming your spouse or significant other for the things that are wrong with your love life? Stop finding fault, focus on yourself, and fix what you don't like about you. Allow your inner strength and joy to be at the heart of who you are. Recognize your own goodness and you'll be able to focus on his goodness, too, rather than his faults.

277. Serve Your Lover Coffee in Bed

A steamy cup of coffee that you can sip in bed before you crawl out in the morning is a treat to be savored. Put the coffee pot on a timer before you go to bed. In the morning place a couple of cups of coffee on a tray, pour the steamy, fragrant brew into the cups, and carry the tray to your bedroom. Serve your lover his and then crawl back in bed and sip yours. You might discover that the coffee becomes less interesting as you become more awake and realize how refreshed and ready you are to enjoy each other.

278. Don't Engage in Casual, Unprotected Sex

Use protection to safeguard your health when having sex, especially if you have sex with multiple partners. Sexually transmitted diseases (STDs), such as genital herpes, chlamydia, gonorrhea, and syphilis are easily spread from one person to another through unprotected sex. The spread of HIV/AIDS has predominantly been due to unprotected sex and the sharing of needles. When you engage in protected sex, you safeguard your own health and that of your sexual partner. Enjoy your lifestyle, be safe, and stay healthy.

279. Take a Second Honeymoon

A second honeymoon is a wonderful way to jump-start a flagging sexual relationship. Go away together—this means away from the house, the kids, your work, and responsibilities to just be with your spouse, doing nothing but getting reacquainted in the bedroom. Order room service, play bedroom games, take romantic walks, hold hands, kiss often, enjoy an expensive meal. Make it a long vacation or just a long weekend, but make certain that it involves lots of love and passion.

280. Buy Some Sexy Lingerie

You don't need an excuse to go underwear shopping. And you don't have to wait until you've lost that last ten or fifteen pounds, either. Even if you've been trying to lose them since the twins were born and now they are about to graduate college. If he's still with you, it's likely he loves you just the way you are. But every girl wants to look her best, so try on some black lacy no-nothings and while you are at it, buy yourself a tube of red lipstick. If you're up for it, put on a little music and do a strip tease for your guy. Ever try to frown while pulling off a thong? Whether it's fun or awkward or both, your effort is bound to put a big smile on your face and that of your partner as well.

281. Get Love on Your Mind

Humans require love to flourish. Love energizes thoughts, empowers individuals to dream and follow their bliss, and enables their efforts to manifest. In his best-selling book, *Think and Grow Rich*, author Napoleon Hill explained that it is by our predominant thoughts that we thrive. Many people might agree that thoughts of love leave a deep "imprint" in the psyche and heart. You become a powerful creator when you learn to transmute negative thoughts into positive ones, for example, anger into appreciation, and then magnetize your thoughts with love. You feel better and look lovelier when love is on your mind and in your heart.

282. See Love as a Powerful Magnet

Love can serve as a powerful magnetizer for manifestation. Here's the way it works. Because of the hormones that are released in your body when you are in love, your thoughts become highly magnetized. When you first fall in love, you may feel crazy and even somewhat obsessive. All you can think about is your beloved. The other person may, in fact, be thinking of you in the exact moment that you are thinking of her. Whether altruistic, romantic, or compassionate, love seeks expression. Passionate love is the driving force behind magnificent works of art, architecture, literature, and music, as well as procreation. Many of us became the expression of our parents' love for each other. Love can draw into your life a romantic partner, meaningful work, pets, and friends.

chapter fourteen

Loosen Up, Literally

283. Understand the Meaning of Flexibility

Flexibility is the ability to move a joint throughout its range of motion. A joint is the place where two or more bones meet; bones are connected by ligaments and tendons, which are connective tissues. Joints allow movement in the body, and flexibility is necessary for efficient movement. Being flexible may also decrease the chance of sustaining muscular injury, soreness, and pain. In other words, when a person lacks flexibility, movement can be limiting, painful, and disabling. Flexibility is essential to your health and a valuable component of your exercise program.

284. Dare to Go Sleeveless Again

Don't like the way your arms look in sleeveless shirts and dresses? Consider weight training to tone and tighten the skin and muscle that may be starting to jiggle. Strength training works because muscles adapt to stress. Your muscles develop strength and endurance when you increase the amount of resistance, work them more often, and push them harder. When your muscles are challenged to lift something heavier than they are used to, they respond by growing stronger to meet the challenge. As the muscle develops, everything tightens and tones. If you want to have arms like the first lady, you have to make a commitment to focus on the upper arm during your workouts.

285. Practice Tai Chi

Flexibility exercises are those that gently stretch muscles, tendons, and ligaments to keep them pliable and mobile. Flexibility exercises include stretching, ballet, yoga, and tai chi. When you are fit and flexible, your body is able to do more with less effort, and that feels great and encourages more activity.

286. Try Yoga's Dead Man's Pose

Doing yoga can help you feel younger and stronger because the postures enable you to strengthen muscles, keep joints flexible, burn calories, and reduce stress levels. If you feel intimidated by attempting a yoga position or asana, try a beginner's pose for ten or fifteen minutes. The dead man's pose (also called the corpse pose) has you lying on your back, hands out to the sides, legs apart. In this position, you can relax and tense the muscles of your body, from head to toe or reverse. If you've got a sedentary job that requires sitting all day behind a computer, stretching often at your desk will enable your body to remain limber. Do yoga at night to calm and center your mind and to release the tensions of the day. You may find you fall to sleep easier and stay asleep longer.

287. Train for a Race with Friends

A major benefit of training with others, especially those of more or less equal ability and experience, is that socializing while running or biking decreases the perceived effort significantly, and that results in a better attitude toward workouts and more effective training. Further, if it's just you scheduled to get in a four-mile run at 5:30 A.M., you might swat that alarm clock and roll over for a bit more sleep. If you are meeting a couple of friends at the park for that early-morning tempo session, you are much more likely to keep to your schedule. Training buddies can be motivators.

288. Develop a Plan to Stay Flexible for Life

Your ability to move easily and perform daily functions is related to your body's flexibility. As you age, muscles and tendons lose their flexibility and strength, and bones become more susceptible to fractures due to shrinkage in size and density. To defy aging, formulate a plan and do exercises to stay flexible throughout your life. For example, bend over, touch your hands on the floor in front of you and use your hands to begin walking forward until your body is stretched out like a board, then walk your hands back and gradually stand upright again. Swing your legs front to back and do the same for your arms. Make small circles with each leg and then large circles. Repeat the same exercise with your arms. Rotate your head right in a smooth and gentle circular motion. Then reverse the rotation. Make these exercises part of your flexibility plan and do them morning and night, or find others that you like to do and stick to doing them to stay flexible.

289. Try Glucosamine

Although glucosamine seems promising for osteoarthritis, not everyone who takes it will experience benefits, and any results take at least six to eight weeks to occur. The usual dosage for osteoarthritis is 1,500 milligrams glucosamine (500 milligrams taken three times a day). If this amount relieves symptoms, the dosage can be gradually decreased. Glucosamine is available as a "hydrochloride" (HCl) and as a "sulfate." Both forms have performed equally well in studies. The glucosamine that's present in supplements is extracted from natural sources such as ground-up crab, lobster, or shrimp shells. Some researchers suggest it isn't necessary to take chondroitin with glucosamine, especially since much of the research on chondroitin used an injectable form, and not pill form. Glucosamine is available in tablet and capsule forms in widely varying dosages.

290. Warm Up Your Muscles Before Exercising

If you run for daily exercise or are in training for a triathlon, you know that your body takes a pounding from the impact of each step. There are many other potentially serious injuries and chronic conditions to deal with, including runner's knee, shin splints, and plantar fasciitis. Perhaps you like swimming and do it competitively. The most common problem for swimmers is in the shoulder area, primarily the rotator cuff. A biker can have problems with the iliotibial band, a long tendon that runs down the side of the leg from the hip to just below the knee. It helps stabilize the knee and can become inflamed from overuse and failure to stretch. No matter what kind of exercise you do, adequate warming and proper stretching can help protect against injury.

291. Stretch Your Muscles in Groups

After a run, concentrate on the glutes (buttocks and hips), the hamstrings, calf muscles, and the plantar fascia (tissues in the foot). For the gluteus muscles, sit on the floor, cross your legs, lean forward, and stretch. For the hamstrings, put your foot on a chair, keeping your leg straight, and lean forward to stretch. Do the same for the other leg. To stretch your calf muscles, put both hands on a wall and extend one leg back, keeping the sole of your foot completely on the ground. Lean in to create some tension in the calf and hold for twenty to thirty seconds. To stretch the plantar fascia in your foot, stand on a step with the ball of your foot and let your heel down.

292. Do the Downward-Facing Dog

A great post-run stretch can be accomplished by using a yoga pose known as downward-facing dog. Make an inverted V with your body, hands and feet planted on the ground or floor and your head down. This accomplishes most of the stretches you need for your backside in one step: glutes, hamstrings, calf muscles, Achilles tendon, lower back, lats (latissimus dorsi), and shoulder muscles.

293. Play Bocce Ball

Some 5,000 years ago, the ancient Egyptians threw balls toward a target in one of the earliest forms of bocce ball. Simply explained, bocce ball is a game in which a team tries to get its four balls closest to the small target ball known as the pallino, which is thrown by the first player to start the game. Today, a game of bocce ball can be played with up to eight players in teams of two or four people. And the sport can be played in the backyard or in a park, on smooth grass or dirt lot, in a hilly area or flat land, or on a formal bocce ball court. People of all sizes, ages, and athletic abilities can play bocce ball, so it's a great choice for getting people together for a little exercise and a whole lot of fun and camaraderie.

294. Spend Five to Fifteen Minutes Daily Strengthening Your Abdomen

A body's strong and sturdy core provides the perfect structure for a flat and toned waistline and figure. Achieving and maintaining a strong core means that you will have to ante up all areas of your life—eating better, sleeping better, and elevating the difficulty and frequency of workouts. Getting rid of belly fat means you will not only look better but feel better—stronger, more flexible, and confident.

295. Consider Training for a Triathlon

If you are relatively new to athletic pursuits, you must understand that it will take your body some time to adjust to the new stresses you will be putting on it by training for a triathlon—a multisport event where you'll run, swim, and bike. Especially where running is concerned, your muscles and tendons will not be used to the strain they are about to experience. Of the three sports you will be undertaking, running will require the most caution. You are about to embark on a journey that could improve and extend your life. People who exercise regularly find it easier to maintain a healthy weight and good blood pressure. They sleep better, live longer, are sick less often, and are more productive at work.

296. Lift Weights

Exercises to increase strength and flexibility include weight lifting (whether through the use of free weights or the kind of weight machines found in most gyms), yoga, and similar stretching activities. Weight-bearing exercises are particularly important for women because they can help prevent the onset of osteoporosis later in life by maintaining bone density before, during, and after menopause. And you don't have to lift weights until you bulge like Mr. Universe; most health specialists say thirty to forty minutes of weight training a week is sufficient to maintain optimum health. Weight training can vastly improve muscle strength, balance, and flexibility—all of which is good for your brain.

297. Don't Overdo Exercise

A study of male Harvard graduates compared longevity rates of major athletes (meaning those who lettered in a particular sport), minor athletes (those who participated but didn't letter), and non-athletes. It was assumed that the major athletes, who presumably exercised the hardest, would have the greatest longevity, but, in fact, it was the minor athletes who lived the longest. What does this mean? Well, for starters, it means that when it comes to life-extending physical activity, moderation is best. There's no need to train like an Olympic athlete, because too much exercise is just as bad as too little. The key is to strengthen and maintain your body's systems, not abuse them through an excessive physical regimen. If you feel pain, you may be working too hard. Slow down and listen to your body.

298. Alternate Workouts When Weightlifting

A well-rounded exercise regimen should strengthen muscles, benefit the heart and lungs, and build endurance. For optimum results, alternate weight training, aerobics, and circuit training. Reliance on only one form of exercise will not benefit your entire body. *Vary your activities to ensure a complete workout.* Weightlifting strengthens your muscles and may help you lose belly fat; you'll also need some cardiovascular activity, such as aerobics, to benefit your heart and lungs—and thus your circulatory system and blood flow to your brain.

299. Hire, or Consult, a Personal Trainer

If you have trouble staying motivated, a personal trainer can be extremely beneficial. In addition to making sure you exercise regularly, she can show you how to perform your workout for maximum advantage. Most gyms have staff that will create the exercise regimen that's best for you and help you through it. This ensures that you are exercising correctly and at the proper pace. If you can afford a personal trainer, she will encourage you to commit to your routine and to push yourself just a wee bit harder—all of which is good for your brain.

300. Practice Pilates

By emphasizing the importance of the mind/body connection in attaining physical fitness, Joseph Pilates married critical elements of Eastern and Western philosophies. Westerners approach health and fitness as a scientific function of maintaining and nurturing the body's muscles, bones, and circulatory and digestive systems.

Eastern philosophies place much more importance on the development of mental and spiritual powers in the pursuit of pure health. Pilates students approach each movement with focus and determination, and they engage body and mind equally in each physical endeavor. Pilates is a conditioning program designed to work the whole body—including your brain—simultaneously and uniformly. Joseph Pilates created his exercises with the intention "that each muscle may cooperatively and loyally aid in the uniform development of all our muscles. Developing minor muscles naturally helps to strengthen major muscles." As a result, every muscle is developed in every movement.

301. Do Yoga Stretches and Postures

Yoga is an ancient Indian method of exercise designed to "yoke" body and mind that involves specific postures, breathing exercise, and meditation. It provides an excellent fitness activity on its own and also makes the perfect complement to other fitness activities because it increases strength, flexibility, circulation, posture, and overall body condition. Practicing yoga is great for people who have a hard time slowing down (you'll learn how great it feels and how important it is to move your body with slow control) and for people who have difficulty engaging in high-impact or fast-paced exercise. You can adapt your routine to your own fitness level to make it decidedly low impact and among the more perfect stress management exercises. Its original purpose was to gain control over the body and bring it into a state of balance in order to free the mind for spiritual contemplation. Yoga can help you to master your body so that it doesn't master you.

302. Try Herbs for Arthritis Pain and Stiffness

When your joints hurt and feel stiff, it's difficult to do the stretching necessary to feel loose and limber. If the problem is arthritis, there are herbs that some people have found beneficial for pain relief. There are two main types of arthritis: osteoarthritis (OA), which is characterized by pain and swelling of the joints, generally due to wear and tear, and rheumatoid arthritis (RA), which is characterized by the inflammation of many joints and requires professional treatment. Rheumatism is a general term for any muscle pain; lumbago is lower-back pain. Symptoms often worsen in damp weather. The key symptoms include stiffness and joint pain, swollen or deformed joints, hot or burning sensations in joints, and creaking sounds in joints. Angelica is a warming and stimulating herb effective for "cold" types of osteoarthritis and rheumatism. Devil's claw has a potent and anti-inflammatory action that has been compared to cortisone. It's better for osteoarthritis and degenerative conditions than for rheumatoid arthritis. Bogbean is a cleansing, cooling, and anti-inflammatory herb useful for "hotter" types of arthritis and for muscle pain. White willow is rich in salicylates, which are anti-inflammatories that cool hot joints; it's especially useful for the pain associated with the acute phases of arthritis and for muscle pain.

303. Buy the Best Herbs You Can Find

If you want to use herbs to feel better, whether for helping your body have less pain or to enhance your mood or increase your stamina, whenever possible, buy fresh herbs that are organically grown or wild crafted (grown in their natural habitat). When buying fresh-dried herbs, make sure they are grown locally. If buying bulk herbs, test a sample by rubbing some between your fingers to check the smell. Even dried herbs when crushed give off strong evidence of their volatile oils, so potency is easily evident. Buy the best-quality herbs available. Bargain herbs are usually adulterated. More costly products from reputable companies are a better choice because the growing/gathering/preparation/storage phases of the process are supported by experience and quality control.

304. Overcome Your Fears of Injury and Begin Exercising

Exercise is good for you as you age, but few people actually take the time to fit physical activity into their busy schedules. Older people, in particular, are often reluctant to exercise for fear of injuring themselves, yet they need it just as much, if not more, than men and women who are younger. In the older population, exercise keeps the heart and lungs working at full capacity, the muscles well toned, the bones strong, and the immune system in tip-top shape. Exercise also helps maintain mental clarity and, when done in a group setting, allows you to remain socially active. Replace your fear of injury with the expectation of feeling better and being healthier.

chapter fifteen

Avoid Contaminants and Pollutants

305. Understand the Pesticides, Chemicals, and Additives in Your Food

Unless you are buying organic and pesticide-free products, you may be getting unwanted ingredients in your food. Commercial growers have to manage pest populations and usually use pesticides to do it. Meats and milk can contain antibiotics and hormones. For example, a pellet inserted in a young heifer's ear can release hormones throughout her life and result in weight gain and higher milk production. Both translate to increased income for farmers. In high concentrations, such pesticides, antibiotics, hormones, and other additives can be harmful to your health. The same is true for exposure to lower amounts, but over an extended period of time. To become informed, read food labels. Shop organic. Or, grow your own food.

306. Detoxify Your Body and Brain

If you suspect that you may have been exposed to dangerous fumes or toxic chemicals, consult a doctor for a thorough analysis and treatment. To cleanse your brain (and your body) of common toxins, such as pollutants or household chemicals, you can try: flaxseed, licorice root, ginseng, ginkgo biloba, aloe vera, grapefruit pectin, papayas, slippery elm bark, alfalfa, peppermint, and ginger tea. You can take capsules or use the ingredients to make tea. You can also drink lemon water, exercise strenuously, take a sauna, get a vigorous massage, and eat a high-fiber cleansing diet. Deep-breathing exercises, in clean environments, will infuse your brain with fresh oxygen. When it comes to minimizing food contaminants, wash all fruits and vegetables thoroughly.

307. Limit Mercury in Your Diet

Research has shown that exposing nerve cells to mercury causes the formation of neurofibrillar tangles and amyloid plaques, often present in Alzheimer's cases. Dr. Haley, a Canadian researcher, reported in a 2001 issue of *NeuroReport* that "Seven of the characteristic markers that we look for to distinguish Alzheimer's disease can be produced in normal brain tissues, or cultures of neurons, by the addition of extremely low levels of mercury. In addition, research [in 1998] has shown that Alzheimer's patients have at least three times higher blood levels of mercury than controls." Dr. William R. Markesbery, director of the Sanders-Brown Center on Aging at the University of Kentucky, found in 1990 that Alzheimer's patients' brain tissue had almost double the concentration of mercury as that of patients who died of all other causes.

308. Avoid Exposure to Toxic Environmental Substances

The concept that environmental substances can make people sick is not new. In fact, it was first proposed in the fourth century B.C. by the Greek physician Hippocrates, who suggested that illness could result from air contaminated by a variety of wastes, including the decay of dead plants and animals. The ancient Romans also understood this concept, noting the potential for disease from exposure to environmental toxins such as mercury, lead, and even asbestos.

309. Know the Routes of Exposure to Toxic Substances

Toxic substances can enter the body through the skin, gastrointestinal tract, and lungs. The skin is your first line of defense in protecting the inside of the body from the outside environment. Skin is tough and offers very good protection from most pollutants, but it's not perfect. Harmful agents can enter the bloodstream if the protective layer of waxy liquid on the skin's surface is broken or dissolved. Wear sufficient protection when working with potentially dangerous chemicals, such as cleaning products, pesticides, and solvents. The gastrointestinal tract protects your internal organs from harmful agents that are ingested. Exposure can occur when soluble compounds are consumed, absorbed, and then taken into the cells. The lungs are the most important—and the most vulnerable—route of exposure to environmental toxins. Potentially dangerous airborne agents can be deposited in the lungs and, if soluble, absorbed into the bloodstream. Smokers are at particular risk because their lungs have already taken a beating.

310. Be Aware of Water Contamination

Water is essential for human life; without it, you can die within days. Water is known as the "universal solvent" because of its amazing ability to pick up other substances after the briefest of exposures. As a result, pure water—that is, water consisting only of H_2O—does not exist in nature. All water has something else in it. Water's ability to attract other chemicals is vital to your very survival. You depend on it to transport nutrients to cells and carry away cellular wastes, and some minerals found naturally in water, such as calcium, magnesium, and iron, are important to cellular survival. But when the water you drink picks up pollutants, problems occur.

311. Exercise Caution in Drinking Water from Unknown Sources

Some of the most worrisome and controversial organic water pollutants are chlorination by-products known as trihalomethanes (THMs), which result when chlorine—one of the most common water disinfectants—reacts with naturally occurring organic matter such as dead plants. The most dangerous THM is chloroform, which is believed to cause cancer in humans. Another organic water pollutant of concern is the family of chlorinated hydrocarbons, which are widely used as industrial solvents. These chemicals are often found in industrial effluents and are frequently discharged into rivers and lakes, where they can contaminate drinking supplies by soaking through the soil into groundwater. Individuals living near toxic waste sites, landfills, and even military bases are most at risk of chlorinated hydrocarbon contamination. The health risk from exposure to chlorinated hydrocarbons is substantial. In high doses, the chemicals can damage the nervous system, liver, and kidneys, and there is some evidence that they also can cause cancer.

312. Avoid Contact with Heavy Metals

Heavy metals are elements, such as lead, mercury, and cadmium, that can be quite bad for your health should they be found in high concentrations in drinking water. Heavy metals can leach into water supplies from a variety of different sources. The most common is aging landfills, which can dump heavy metals into nearby groundwater. However, heavy metals can also find their way into municipal water supplies when dumped into sewers by metal-finishing companies, or into your home tap water via corroded pipes. Of the latter, lead, cadmium, and copper are the most frequently detected.

313. Know the Dangers of Heavy Metals to Your Health

In addition to interfering with a variety of body processes, heavy metals can damage the brain, nervous system, and kidneys, and cause male infertility. Fetuses and infants are particularly sensitive to the effects of heavy metals, particularly lead. Indeed, lead poses one of the greatest health threats when it comes to your water. In high doses, this metal, which once was commonly used in household plumbing, can cause severe brain damage and even death; in low doses, it can cause nerve system damage in still-developing fetuses, infants, and children. The most common effects include learning disabilities and hyperactive behavior.

314. Understand the Health Threat of Radon

This naturally occurring radioactive gas is formed when uranium decays; it poses a very serious health threat, especially when it gets into drinking water. In fact, many environmental experts believe waterborne radon may be responsible for more cancer deaths than all other drinking-water contaminants combined. According to the Environmental Protection Agency, inhaled indoor radon results in between 5,000 and 20,000 lung cancer deaths annually. Most of these deaths are the result of radon gas rising up from the ground and accumulating in homes through cracks in basements and foundations. However, a small percentage—perhaps up to 1,800 deaths per year—are believed to be caused by radon in household water. The health hazard is not from the consumption of contaminated water but from radon dissolved in the water escaping into the indoor air when water is sprayed in showers and washing machines.

315. Know If Nitrate Pollution Is a Problem Where You Live

Drinking water typically provides around 1 percent of a person's daily intake of nitrates, with the rest coming from vegetables. But in some areas of the country, water supplies from private wells in farming areas may contain dangerously high levels of these chemicals, which usually result from the use of chemical fertilizers and manure. However, water from leaking septic tanks can also contaminate groundwater with nitrates. Those most at risk of nitrate exposure are infants younger than six months old. Consuming formula made with water contaminated with nitrates can result in a dangerous condition known as methemoglobinemia, in which the blood has difficulty transporting oxygen. Symptoms include shortness of breath and weakness.

316. Get Your Tap Water Tested

If you use a municipal water supply that services more than 500 people, the utilities department is required by federal law to test its water regularly and make the findings of those tests available to the public free of charge. So the first thing you should do if you have any questions regarding your drinking water is contact your local water company and ask for the last complete analysis. It's important to note that this analysis will tell you the quality of the water when it left the treatment plant—not necessarily as it pours out of your household tap. As a result, your household water may contain higher levels of lead, for example, than the analysis reports because lead has leached into your water through municipal or household pipes on its way from the treatment plant to your faucet. If you are concerned, have a private lab test your tap water.

317. Understand the Health Risks of Breathing Polluted Air

Anyone who has lived in an area where smog alerts are common knows the symptoms of breathing dirty air; they include an irritated throat, respiratory problems, watery eyes, and so forth. Known as "transient ailments," these symptoms may also include skin rashes, headaches, nausea, and dizziness. However, chronic exposure to outdoor air pollution, such as that experienced by people living in overcrowded urban areas or factory towns, can also lead to a variety of dangerous chronic health conditions such as emphysema, bronchitis, asthma, and even cancer.

318. Check Your Home Air Quality

If you think that staying home all day will protect you from air pollution, you're wrong. Because most homes are sealed tight due to the use of air conditioners, many potentially harmful substances cannot escape into the atmosphere, so instead they build up inside our homes until, very often, they reach levels higher than air pollutants outdoors! Some indoor air pollutants, such as radon gas or airborne mold, occur naturally; others, such as tobacco smoke, are the result of lifestyle choices. Many different indoor pollutants are emitted by material possessions, such as formaldehyde fumes from carpeting and processed wood, and carbon monoxide from poorly vented gas stoves and heating units. There's no way to escape it; modern living often means polluted air.

319. Never Remove Asbestos Yourself

The use of asbestos as a building material was banned in 1974, but so much of the stuff was used as fireproofing in construction prior to the ban that it is still considered a serious indoor air pollutant—and rightly so. Asbestos fibers can cause lung cancer and other serious respiratory problems, including asbestosis and bronchogenic carcinoma. Asbestos poses no hazard as long as it remains intact. However, should it be torn apart during construction or demolition, or simply start to break down from age, fibers can be released into the air and eventually inhaled. If your house was constructed before the 1974 asbestos construction ban, there is a considerable chance that it contains asbestos in some form. If so, do not try to remove it yourself! Only qualified professionals should remove it.

320. Stay Away from Secondhand Tobacco Smoke

The dangers of smoking—and of inhaling secondhand smoke—become evident when you understand the number and type of toxic substances released when tobacco is burned. One of the most worrisome is benzene, an extremely harmful substance that is believed to be responsible for many cases of leukemia. The levels of benzene can be extremely high in a closed home with many smokers, and anyone breathing such polluted air faces serious health risks over time.

321. Use Hand Sanitizer

Make your mother proud by washing your hands often and practicing the good hygiene rituals she taught when you were a child. Do your part to avoid spreading germs. Hand sanitizers come in small bottles that can go into a purse or a pocket. If you can't wash your hands, use the sanitizer (generally, it dries without the necessity of wiping) before consuming food. You can even put a glob on a napkin and wipe down your eating area if the restaurant where you are dining doesn't use cloth or paper table cloths that are customarily changed before you are seated. Use of a hand sanitizer can help you stay healthy and keep germs at a distance.

chapter sixteen

Strengthen Your Social Network

322. Understand the Importance of Social Connections

During the earliest days of human existence, a group of individuals, working together, could stalk and kill large prey that would provide food for several days. Groups also provided protection from larger predators and marauding invaders. Consequently, loose groups of primitive humans banded together to form organized tribes, which eventually led to collectives, towns, and cities. This primitive social interaction was important for physical survival and still is today. Collectively we provide food, goods, and services for the survival and comfort of everyone. But more important are the emotional and psychological benefits that come from human communication and interaction. Being with friends and loved ones makes you feel good emotionally and that, in turn, benefits your health, your aging process, and how you look and feel.

323. Build a Strong Support System for Your Life

The definition of social contact or social support varies among people and organizations but is generally considered to be the belief by individuals that they are cared for, loved, and part of a network of mutual obligations. This support system is instilled and confirmed by caring communication with family, friends, and others and has been shown to protect us from a wide variety of stress-related physical and mental conditions ranging from arthritis to depression. Studies have also shown that people with strong social support require less pain medication following surgery, recover more rapidly, and take better care of themselves following illness or hospitalization. A strong social support system is characterized by the following:

- Strong social support encourages healthy living and promotes prompt medical care. Our friends and family look out for us, just as we look out for them, and often become deeply involved when we get sick. Their concern encourages us to seek medical care when necessary, and we recover faster as a result.
- Friends and family are often impromptu "doctors," directly caring for us when we get sick. Without this assistance, we might stay sick longer or become increasingly ill.
- Our circle of close family and friends encourages a certain degree of conformity. Very often, this includes conforming to a relatively healthful lifestyle. For example, if few of our friends smoke or drink, we are less likely to smoke or drink. Similarly, if the majority of our friends and family engage in a healthful activity, such as golf or tennis, we too are likely to pursue that activity.
- Friendship and loving support can actually boost our immune system, making us more resistant to illness. Positive emotions can actually stimulate our body to prevent or fight illness, a phenomenon known as the mind-body connection.

324. Go on a Date with Someone Younger Than You

Put yourself back into circulation. Meet new people by trying some of the newest dating strategies. Online dating sites have proliferated in recent years. Some charge a fee and some do not. Increasingly, speed dating is an interesting option utilized by upwardly mobile young professionals. Back in the day, people thought of matchmakers as belonging within only certain cultures, but more recently matchmakers have gone mainstream and have found the web and the Yellow

Pages perfect venues for advertising their services: namely, to help you find Ms. or Mr. Right. If you seek a companion for your life and haven't yet found one that's a keeper, don't give up. You have more options and tools than ever for finding that perfect someone. And while you're at it, be open to dating someone younger than you.

325. Help a Friend Prune Her Roses

Spin your love of roses and caring for them into an opportunity for social networking—an important factor in longevity. For example, work in the garden of a friend. Gardening with your friend can strengthen your relationship with her and provide ample opportunities to learn more about her life, garden, and plants. Each time you are out in the garden with her clipping off spent rose blooms or cutting out overlapping canes, you are not only nurturing the plants but building an enduring friendship, and that's good for both of you.

326. Ask a Neighbor to Show You How to Build Birdhouses

It's easier to form a bond with someone by asking him to show you how to do something that he loves doing. For example, if your neighbor loves gardening and has successfully grafted several new varieties of apples onto a tree in his yard, ask him to show you how. Or, if another neighbor makes birdhouses, show an interest in her artistic creations. Perhaps the lady on the corner makes jewelry to sell on eBay. Maybe you know how to do something that your neighbors don't and you could demonstrate your hobby, craft, or skill to them.

chapter seventeen
Renew Your Spirit

331. Go Silent for a Day

The word for observing silence in Sanskrit is "mauna," and involves quieting the chatter of the mouth and also the mind. The path of silence is an ancient method of spiritual renewal. Observing silence enhances concentration. Some monasteries and novitiates permit visitors to join their communities for personal retreats, and during the span of the retreat (often one to several days), silence is observed. If you find such a practice difficult, but would like to try it, search out a supervised silent retreat in a religious or spiritual center.

332. Let Love Flow from You

Love, some say, is itself a vibration. Left unimpeded, love can flow easily between humans. But when love meets resistance in the form of deep-seated selfishness, fear, angst, and a need to control, its flow becomes as impeded or erratic as surely as when a stream hits a narrow gorge or tumbles onto a craggy beach filled with boulders. When you block giving or receiving love, you are thwarting your opportunity to be nourished as intended by the heart of the Divine. Open yourself to the inflowing love from the Source of your being, permit it to spiritually renew you, and then let it flow from you into your relationships and onward into the world.

333. Walk a Spiritual Path or Road

Some paths have been trod by pilgrims seeking spiritual renewal for centuries, for example, Jerusalem's Via Dolorosa, or the pilgrim's path leading to Mecca, or the Bodhi Tree in Bodhgaya, India, where

Buddha became enlightened. Perhaps there's a spiritual trail or road in your part of the world. If not, consider walking along one of the ancient routes that spiritual pilgrims through the centuries have trod. Or, take a walk in nature and get reacquainted with the feeling of wonder and renewal all around you.

334. Attract Healing with Belief

Practicing your faith is especially important if you are in need of healing. In such a time of need, spiritual renewal is often also needed. It is often difficult to assess whether or not a chronically ill person has experienced a miraculous cure. Certainly doctors can attest to the recovery but explaining such a sudden (sometimes instantaneous) recovery in someone who has been diagnosed with a chronic affliction or terminal disease can be impossible. Still, many people do recover through the power of their faith and unshakable belief that they will become healthy again. When they have such faith and belief of having excellent health, they are setting up a powerful force for attracting recovery.

335. Be Mindful of What You Sow

The karmic law or the law of retribution states that what you sow, you reap; also, what you send out comes back. What you think about most is what you draw into your life experience. Throughout an average day in your life, are you thinking lovingly of the welfare of others or falling into a pattern of criticizing others for everything that makes you unhappy and stressed out? According to the tenets of Hinduism, your thoughts are as powerful as a spoken word. Words, like your actions, are creating your karma and when the elements are ripe for those words and actions to bear fruit (whether good or bad), they will.

336. Know Your Spiritual Strengths and Weaknesses

Spiritual well-being comes about as a result of living a clean and decent life, observing nonviolence, caring for your family, performing your work and worldly duties, and practicing your religion or spiritual tradition. It is also important to show respect for all life and reverence toward that which is considered sacred. Work for change from the inside out and try to turn your spiritual weaknesses into spiritual strengths.

337. Engage in Action Without Action

There is a concept in Taoism called "not doing," or *wu-wei.* In a discussion of generosity of spirit, wu-wei has a place because of its emphasis on living life from the spirit, expressing harmony and love in all you do. The power behind wu-wei's "action without action" is synchronicity. When you set forth an intent or desire in your mind and are harmoniously aligned with the energy of the Tao, your power, invisible and strong, works with the laws of the universe. From that place of strength, you will feel renewed, invigorated, and full of hope, optimism, and expectation.

338. Read a Book about Angels

When you feel the weight of the world upon your shoulders, read about angels, those celestial companions that many of the great religious traditions of the world have placed between humans and the Supreme Being. If you haven't already, notice how images of angels are everywhere. When you feel as if your world is full of challenges and difficulties, believing in a higher power and angelic helpers might lift your spirits. Find something that resonates with your beliefs in order to help your heart to return to that inner oasis of peace and love. Try to feel joyful again.

339. Hang Wind Chimes for Their Soothing Sounds

Wind chimes, according to the ancient Chinese tradition of Feng Shui, can restore the movement of energy to places where it has become stagnant. A soft melodious chiming sound can soothe a weary spirit. Hanging wind chimes in your home or garden can be especially effective in creating sacred space. Whether the chimes are made of hollow bamboo, metal tubes, or crystal bars, they can provide a soft ambient sound to any place where you sit to summon the power of the universe to reenergize body and spirit.

340. Remind Yourself That Life Is Cyclic

When you are faced every day with the realities of life, much of it negative, keep reminding yourself that life is rhythmic, cyclic, and always evolving. It's difficult not to notice repetition and renewal going on all the time. Just as darkness comes at the end of each day, so also the dawn arrives to spread light over the land. Just as plants must die at the end of their life cycle, the seeds they have dropped will emerge as new plants in the spring. There will always be good times

and bad, feasts and famines, hot summers and cold winters. Whenever you feel stuck or spiritually dry or just plain gloomy, take time to
remind yourself that change is on its way. It's a given.

341. Take a Break from the News

With all the negative messages coming at you every day from myriad directions, you may wonder how you can possibly feel optimistic about anything. Perhaps you have begun to feel disjointed,
trying to hold hopefulness in your heart but at the same time seeing
or hearing news stories about the downward slide of the global
economy, the escalation of armed conflicts that Americans are
fighting, and the emerging stories of the lies that have been told
by financiers and world leaders. A global peace seems ever more
elusive. So how do you find spiritual sustenance and renewal in
such a negative climate? One way might be to take a break from
the news. Turn off the television and radio. Don't click onto Internet
news stories. Stop the daylong bombardment of negativity from
virtually every media outlet. Take a break from the news, and after
a day or two, evaluate just how much of an impact the news has
been having on your sense of well-being.

342. Embrace a Symbol's Esoteric Meaning

There are literally thousands of symbols, from ancient to modern.
Some may have obscure meanings while others are universally
understood. While certain symbols may be associated with myths
and cultural traditions, others hold special meaning only for certain

groups. Some symbols have represented a specific meaning for centuries. However, such symbols may also have other meanings associated with them, depending upon the culture in which they are found. For example, the cross, a sacred symbol for Christians, is also the symbol of earth to the Chinese. Symbols can remind you to let go of worry and to center and anchor yourself in something greater than the self. A symbol can guide you inward to a place of peaceful contemplation, diminishing stress, and restoring a sense of harmony so important in healthful living.

343. Choose a Personal Spiritual Symbol

Spiritual symbols have the power to alter consciousness if they are used for such purpose. For example, perhaps you desire to use a symbol to represent a metaphysical truth or a transcendent state of mind. Consider the Hindu symbol of Aum as a point of reflection. It is believed to be the sound of the cosmic vibration of the universe. The yin/yang symbol that represents the opposite principles of masculine and feminine in Chinese philosophy signifies harmony, balance, and universal fellowship to some people. A dragon or bear image suggests strength and fortitude. What do you need to feel better, healthier, younger, and more beautiful? Find a symbol that addresses those things for you.

344. Root Out Doubt

You can create any dream, including vibrant health, spiritual renewal, or simply a deeper connection with your Creator from the field of infinite potentiality. When you grasp that idea, you can let go of attachment to the outcome. The notion of detachment may be for some a little more difficult concept to grasp. It requires letting go of the attachment to the result or outcome of your desire, your dream. That doesn't mean you have to let go of your intention to manifest something. To be able to detach from an outcome means that you have a deep abiding conviction in your true Self's power to create anything you need, want, or desire.

345. Practice the Law of Attraction

Practitioners of the Law of Attraction believe that it is possible to manifest abundant prosperity, good health, meaningful relationships, and high life satisfaction using that ancient law, so well known today because of recent media hype around it. Focusing your mind on what you want, and being grateful for the blessings you already have, will set up an attraction to draw into your life what you think about. Why not give it a try? What you do with the rest of your life is in your hands. The years ahead might even be better than the years of your youth that you've already lived.

chapter eighteen

Tap the Mind-Body Connection

346. Shift Your Thinking about Aging

Research done over the last few decades has shed tremendous light on how age affects the brain and body and how you can keep your mental faculties sharp regardless of your chronological age. Many common types of mental degeneration are the result of lifestyle choices—how you treat your body and brain—more than age, and very often can be reversed with simple changes in diet, lifestyle, or medication. Believe in anti-aging possibilities, incorporate lifestyle changes, and take proactive steps to keep your brain young and your body fit and healthy regardless of your age.

347. Get a New Attitude about Your Dietary Habits

A lousy diet can be a springboard for a wide variety of age-related problems, including hypertension, heart disease, diabetes, osteoporosis, and even cancer. But a simple change in dietary habits can have a remarkable effect on your health and, in turn, how you age—no matter how old you are when you start. For most people, simply eating less red meat and fatty foods and more fresh vegetables and fruits improves their health. This reduces the amount of cholesterol in your system, gives your body the vitamins and minerals it needs to function well, and packs your system with antioxidants and other anti-aging compounds. In turn, your immune system is strengthened. Your body repels illness and has the nutrients and other elements it needs to repair itself and generate robust health, and that enables you to feel more energetic and have a sense of well-being.

348. Think Positive Thoughts

According to Daniel G. Amen, MD, author of *Making a Good Brain Great,* every thought releases brain chemicals. Positive, happy, hopeful thoughts produce specific chemicals that create a sense of well-being and help your brain function at peak capacity; unhappy, miserable, negative thoughts have the opposite effect, effectively slowing down your brain and even creating depression. When you are angry or depressed, you often frown and scowl, and those facial expressions produce wrinkles. If you tend to focus on negative thoughts, you can dim your brain's capacity to function. It saps the brain of its positive forcefulness. Dr. Amen suggests writing out negative thoughts to dispel their power over your brain. Replace them with positive commitments, goals, and actions.

349. Daydream a Sexy New You

Psychologists say that daydreaming is good for you because it can stimulate your mind in creative ways, reduce stress, elevate your mood, organize your thinking, stimulate ideas for solutions to problems, and help you gain new perspectives on troubling issues. Picture yourself as looking fabulous and feeling healthy, young at heart, and fully engaged in life. The more specific you are about what you want—and want to become—the better your ability to manifest that vision of a beautiful, healthy new you.

350. Know That Optimal Health Is Possible

Experts in the emerging field of mind-body medicine say that science is beginning to accept what many of our grandmothers have always known—a psychological link exists between the mind and the body. Consider the possibility that physical well-being is rooted in wanting to feel good. People who believe that they can have optimal health are more likely to obtain such results than people who don't feel that way. Conversely, a person's mental state might also dictate his susceptibility to disease. So, could it be that the body and brain are hard-wired in a way that dictates health or illness? Use your mind to imagine optimal health. Make up autosuggestions to reinforce your imagery to maintain a strong immune system that will fight off age-related diseases.

351. Try Some Biofeedback

Biofeedback, once considered an alternative therapy that places emphasis on the intimate links between the mind, body, and behavior is widely accepted today as a preventative modality to thwart or disrupt illness, injury, and disease. Biofeedback falls into the discipline of mind-body medicine. Not relying purely on your state of physical health but also considering emotional, spiritual, social, and behavioral factors that can affect your health, mind-body medicine uses biofeedback as one intervention. Use biofeedback to deal with outside influences on your health and well-being. Such influences could include stress and environmental factors.

352. Understand How Your Emotions Affect Your Body

When you are feeling stress, grief, or debilitating worry and anxiety in some area of your life, your body can react in a variety of ways to let you know that there's an emotional imbalance. This response in the body is commonly referred to as the mind-body connection. You might suddenly be unable to fall asleep, feel lightheaded, have heart pains or palpitations, become constipated or have diarrhea, gain or lose weight, or develop a stiff neck and tightness in your shoulder muscles. It's just your body's way of telling you that your emotions are affecting the body's normal functioning. Learn stress reduction techniques to stay emotionally healthy, and your body will feel good too.

353. See Yourself as Ageless, Timeless, and Perfect

Stop beating up on yourself over another gray hair, a new or deeper wrinkle, or less than glowing skin. Close your eyes and step away from physical images. Ask yourself how you would feel if you had no idea how old you were. Forget for a moment that you have a body. Be present in your consciousness. For a moment, imagine yourself ageless, ever new, and perfect. Take time every day to just anchor yourself in that place where you stop seeing yourself in a limited way confined to a body in order to perceive yourself in an expansive way. Allow yourself to sense a grander, more spectacular you.

354. Affirm the Unlimited Potential in You

If you think you are powerless to change your life, think again. The body-mind connection is so strong that what a person believes about her health is enough to cause symptoms to appear or improve or disappear. The last is known as the placebo effect: when a person thinks a therapy or drug that contains no medicine will make her better, she will improve just by taking it. Changing your thoughts about the state of your health can enable you to begin feeling stronger. Or, just releasing thoughts about hardships can make them disappear. When you are peaceful, you can draw into your life that which you most ardently desire. But when your mind is polluted with worry you seem to get more of that, don't you? Permit yourself a moment to affirm the unlimited potential in you. Imagine how life will be for you once you let go of obsessive worry and start attracting vibrant health, longevity, prosperity, and serenity.

355. Imagine Your White Blood Cells as Strong Soldiers

Your body responds to messages from the mind. Think of something you want to manifest, for example, the loss of ten pounds, more mental acuity, mastery of some new dance steps, or a stronger immune system so that you rarely, if ever, get sick. Keep visualizing a positive result. Doing so not only enables you to clearly see the outcome you desire, but also helps you create it. How is that possible? According to Dr. Frank Lawlis in *The IQ Answer*, your brain's prefrontal cortex seeks to create what you think you want. Just imagine the possibilities. You could add an extra mile to your morning run by simply seeing it first in your mind. Or, you might visualize your body fighting off a cold by first seeing your white blood cells as ferocious soldiers decimating enemy invaders.

356. Imagine Your Positive Words Hitting Their Mark

Words, poet Emily Dickenson, once wrote, are like boots that walk away, not to be called back. Let your words be carefully chosen, purposefully phrased so that they always carry your intended impact. You don't want to speak in haste, such as in anger or hurtful retaliation, for although you can apologize, you can't call words back once they are spoken. When you discuss your hopes and dreams, positive emotion and passion is the propellant behind the words that you express. Try to convey your thoughts supercharged with belief and emotion and you may find that your words carry a greater and more positive impact than negatively charged language.

357. Undertake a Vision Quest

If you are feeling increasingly fragmented and desire to reconnect with a sense of wholeness or to enhance your own mind-body connection, explore such natural healing alternatives as rolfing, reiki, or reflexology, which involve body work to overcome emotional/psychological/mental issues. Or, try therapies for natural healing such as herbology or aromatherapy. Another option is to undertake a vision quest by spending time in a Native American sweat lodge to cleanse the body and mind, for example. The vision quest is best done out in nature, alone, in quiet. Use the opportunity to commune with a higher power or force to gain a sense of purpose and direction for your life. Done correctly, a vision quest can help you sense the wholeness in the fabric of the universe and yourself as a thread in that fabric.

358. Fix It or Forget It

Do what you can to resolve the stressful situations in your life and stop worrying about those you can't resolve. After all, what's the sense of losing sleep and harming your health dwelling on things over which you have no control? Some people seem better able to invest energy into doing what they can about a problem and, if there's nothing that can be done, they'll just move on. Sometimes we hold on to things too long, thinking there has to be a way to work through every issue, problem, situation, complication, and the like. But the reality is that some things are just unfixable. There's no point in mulling things over endlessly in your mind.

359. Make a Ten-Point List of What Really Matters to You

Millions of people live their lives without a sense of direction. Unless you know what is really important to you and what you want out of life, how are you going to know where you are going, how to get what you want, and what your life purpose is? Think of ten things that are really important to you, for example, family togetherness. Then make each item as specific as possible. Instead of family togetherness, maybe you really mean eating meals together, working on the chores together, or praying together. Refine the ten things on your list until you know exactly what is of primary importance to you. These are the things that will make you happiest.

360. Tense and Release for Peak Performance

Actors, musicians, public speakers, and people taking important examinations know that preparing for a major audition, recital, speaking engagement, or test can play havoc on your body due to rising levels of tension and stress. Tension and stress can also compromise your immune system. An acne breakout or onset of a cold is the last thing you need when you are getting ready for an important appearance. To lighten up and manage the pressure for a peak performance, practice tension and release for each muscle group, in turn, starting with your feet. After you are relaxed, visualize a past event where you have given an outstanding performance. Then visualize details of the upcoming event and see yourself performing at your highest ability.

361. Write a List of What You Feel Grateful for Today

Focus on what you love about your life and your emotional brain fires up. Write out five things you're grateful for today. Focus on what it is about your life that makes you feel young and happy. This trains your brain to focus on the love and pleasant experiences that you have had and are having. You'll effectively create a positive groove in your brain that will generate ripple effects in your life. Your gratitude for the blessings in your life helps you feel happier and more positive—and those feelings of gratitude and joy enable you to attract more.

362. Try Hypnosis for Pain

Ample anecdotal and scientific data exists to support the use of hypnosis to lessen the pain of childbirth, bone marrow aspiration, and burn debridement, among other painful conditions. Other health conditions for which the use of hypnosis has proved beneficial include ulcers, cancer, migraines, and asthma. Discuss the use of hypnosis with your physician or health practitioner. Many New Age bookstores and healing centers carry self-hypnosis tapes and CDs that you can try. You might also make your own self-hypnosis tape by reading a script you've created and setting it to quiet instrumental music.

363. Use Guided Imagery to Lessen the Anxiety of Medical Treatments

If you must undergo a medical treatment, whether it is for the removal of an ingrown toenail or something more serious, consider guided imagery to lesson your anxiety. You will use your imagination or your "mind's eye" to see the part of your body that needs healing while listening to instructions guiding you to visualize a positive image or imagine the optimal outcome. For example, listening to a guided visualization CD or audiotape through headphones, you'll be instructed to relax and then to visualize yourself somewhere in a safe place. The narrator will lead you through one or more scenarios that help you feel less fearful and more confident in dealing with anxiety, pain, and stress of a treatment as well as any associated side effects.

364. Take a Serenity Break to Clear Your Mind

If you want to increase your ability to focus attention on something, take an hour serenity break. Don't use it to check mail messages on your BlackBerry, tweet on your Twitter account, or check stock updates. Instead, take a walk among the flowers, meditating some-place where you won't be interrupted, or enjoying the quiet beauty of a sanctuary like a Japanese tea garden. Scientists who study the mind-body connection say that we are increasingly distracted, thanks, in part, to modern technology and a proliferation of tech-nological gadgets vying for our attention. You can increase your mind's ability to pay attention by giving it a quiet serenity break. Meditation is especially good because it calms the mind, focuses on the present, and allows the body to release tension.

365. Get Stress Inoculation Training

Have you ever been through an extremely stressful situation from which you felt you were never going to recover? It's not unusual for people who have gone through traumatic events to be haunted by the memory of it and to have their bodies respond with symptoms of anxiety, apprehension, and fear. A treatment known as stress inoculation training offers coping strategies and can also be used as a preventative against future triggers or stressors. The treatment has been shown effective in treating post-traumatic stress syn-drome as well as asthma, hypertension, and anger management. Give it a try if you suffer from post-traumatic stress or if stressors in your environment are limiting your ability to feel great or to achieve optimum results in competitive events.

Index

About the Authors

Meera Lester received her training as a respiratory therapist at the University of Missouri and subsequently worked for a dozen years in intensive care units and emergency rooms of several metropolitan hospitals on the West Coast before embarking upon a career as a writer. She cofounded Writers Connection, a San Francisco Bay Area writers organization, and directed its annual Selling to Hollywood screenwriting conferences that attracted writers worldwide. Her work garnered her letters of commendation from Senator Dianne Feinstein and the City of Los Angeles for her contributions to the film industry. An internationally published author, Lester has written hundreds of articles and over a dozen books, including *365 Ways to Live Happy* and *The Everything*® *Law of Attraction Book*.

Carolyn Dean, MD, is a medical doctor and a naturopathic doctor. She attended Dalhousie Medical School in Nova Scotia, Canada, and Ontario Naturopathic College, and sits on the board of the Canadian College of Naturopathic Medicine in Toronto. Dr. Dean is the health expert for *www.yeastconnection.com,* has been featured in their "Ask the Experts" column, and is a regular guest on *The View*. She is the author of *The Everything*® *Alzheimer's Book*, and lives in City Island, New York.